Palgrave Studies in the History of Childhood

Series Editors:

George Rousseau
University of Oxford, UK

Laurence Brockliss
University of Oxford, UK

Aims of the Series

Palgrave Studies in the History of Childhood is the first of its kind to historicise childhood in the English-speaking world; at present no historical series on children/childhood exists, despite burgeoning areas within Child Studies. The series aims to act both as a forum for publishing works in the history of childhood and a mechanism for consolidating the identity and attraction of the new discipline.

More information about this series at
http://www.springer.com/series/14586

Steven J. Taylor

Child Insanity in England, 1845–1907

palgrave
macmillan

Steven J. Taylor
University of Leicester
Leicester, United Kingdom

Palgrave Studies in the History of Childhood
ISBN 978-1-349-95606-7 ISBN 978-1-137-60027-1 (eBook)
DOI 10.1007/978-1-137-60027-1

Printed on acid-free paper

This Palgrave Macmillan imprint is published by Springer Nature
The registered company is Macmillan Publishers Ltd. London
The registered company address is: The Campus, 4 Crinan Street, London, N1 9XW, United Kingdom

For
The Boys

Acknowledgements

The intellectual premise for this piece of work was conceived while working as a teacher of history at a secondary school in Northamptonshire. However, it did not become a reality until a meeting with Professor Steven King at the University of Leicester on a snowy December day in 2010. Steve listened to my ideas and helped refine some of my, what were then lofty, goals. His knowledge, wit, and good humour guided me successfully through the PhD process and this work would never have reached the point of publication without him. The research is better developed and more lucid for Steve's input than I imagined it could ever be. His tolerance of my writing habits and style, so different from his own, knew no bounds. I am truly appreciative of his supervision and friendship and hope to be able to work with him again in the future.

The analysis itself was completed following an extensive period of archival research. During this time I spent countless hours talking to archivists and asking questions that, no matter how banal, they answered dutifully. These individuals deserve a special thank you. As historians we rely on their archival expertise and without them our work would be impossible. It saddens me that many of them are no longer in post as a result of budget cuts, most of which politically imposed, following the financial crisis of 2008. Not only was their subject knowledge of great benefit, but their physical strength, hauling around the large leather-bound casebooks that have survived from asylums, was also appreciated. With hindsight, their good humour and tolerance for my demands was above and beyond the call of duty. To all of the archivists that helped me along the way—I owe you a huge debt.

I also need to offer my gratitude to those who have commented or asked questions about my work at conferences, seminars, and workshops where I have presented. While too numerous to name individually they have helped to mould my thinking and conclusions, and for this they deserve a special mention. For reading drafts of this research I would like to thank Elizabeth Hurren, Rob Ellis, Keith Snell and Peter Bartlett for their time and invaluable feedback on my work. Additionally, the comments from Hilary Marland, who examined my PhD, have been instrumental in shaping the argument and direction of the analysis that follows. I owe Annmarie Valdes more chocolate cake than one can imagine! She has dutifully read chapters and offered advice throughout the writing stages of this book and without her motivational tweets from across the pond I may never have finished. Also I must thank Emily Russell and Rowan Milligan at Palgrave Macmillan for their tolerance, help, and support, and Laurence Brockliss and George Rousseau, the series editors for their input and guidance. For the shortcomings that remain, I alone am responsible.

On a personal level there are a numerous people that I need to acknowledge. Family members have been a constant source of enthusiasm and guidance. My parents, Mag and Rob, have been supportive throughout and have acted as sounding boards, financial consultants, and childminders on numerous occasions. Similarly Bec and Gareth have often stepped in when the need for childcare has been at its most urgent and I hope to now return the favour as the pitter patter of tiny feet are imminent. It is also important that I pay tribute to those who were here at the beginning of this journey but sadly did not see its conclusion. To Mick and, my grandmother, Sheila, you are missed every day and your encouragement and support is appreciated.

Without Lou this book would never have happened and I would most likely still be stuck away in a secondary school classroom somewhere—to her I owe a giant thank you and probably an even bigger apology! Lastly, I turn to the constant sources of energy and distraction in my life—*the boys*. Their good humour has helped me to focus and unwind after periods of archival fatigue and writer's block. At times they have acted as research assistants (only semi-effective) and I have fond memories of teaching them to read using numerous scholarly texts (again, only semi-effective). They are my inspiration and motivation and it is to them that this work is dedicated.

Contents

List of Abbreviations

BCA	Birmingham City Archive
BMJ	British Medical Journal
BLAS	Bedford and Luton Archive Service
GMCRO	Greater Manchester County Record Office
LMA	London Metropolitan Archive
LRO	Lancashire Record Office
NRO	Northamptonshire Record Office

List of Figures

List of Tables

CHAPTER 1

Introduction

The nineteenth-century pauper lunatic asylum conjures a distinct image in the modern imagination—often more haunting and terrifying than what was the reality. Nevertheless, horror stories of asylums and their lunatic residents have become embedded in cultural memory. Were children patients of these institutions? The answer is yes, but their ubiquity, nature of illness, period of confinement, and recovery rates are all issues yet to be explored. Because of our modern perspective the presence of children is surprising to many, but the number of people suffering from insanity in the nineteenth century exploded and the young were not exempt. The vast majority of the insane, both young and old, came from the lower echelons of society and by 1871 they were considered a distinct enough population to be recorded on the decennial census. Defined in medical terms, this social group was considered threatening to productive society and sufferers were kept in asylums for care, treatment, or regulation, depending on your view.

This book examines the experiences of 'insane' children across the period 1845 to 1907. The start point being the introduction of legislation establishing asylums and making the confinement of the insane compulsory, and the end being the creation of the School Medical Service that changed medical and educational approaches towards children. As well as exploring childhood encounters with asylums, the chapters that follow also use the child as a historical prism to observe a broad range of medical, welfare, and status issues. Such issues were exemplified by the

S.J. Taylor, *Child Insanity in England, 1845-1907*, Palgrave Studies in the History of Childhood, DOI 10.1007/978-1-137-60027-1_1

Children's Act 1908 that signified a new legislative outlook towards the young. While this just falls outside of the period in question, the 1908 Act sought more than any other previous legislation to protect the child as an entity separate from the adult world. It declared that children were no longer to be incarcerated in adult prisons, prohibited children from purchasing tobacco and entering public houses, and gave local authorities the power to keep them outside of workhouses. In many ways, by the end of the period examined here, childhood was being conceptualised in a modern sense. A core facet of this construction was the protection of the child and here we explore their entry/admission into spaces of care designed for the vulnerable.

Childhood, evidently, was not a static or objective term and 'insane' children had their social role and status continually defined and shaped by the state throughout the sixty-two years in question. In the early nineteenth century able-bodied children occupied important roles as wage earners in the domestic economies of the working and dependent poor and they were found in both industrial and agricultural work places.[1] As the century progressed, however, the economic importance of the young was gradually eroded by an emotional investment forced upon working families by a professional and increasingly influential middle class.[2] This intrusion was influenced by Romanticist and Evangelical discourses that considered childhood a time of innocence, fun, education, and protection. Exposure to the adult spheres of employment and the wage economy raised anxieties as to the moral and physical well-being of the young. These concerns eventually found expression in numerous Acts of Parliament designed to restrict the working age of children. The first of these, the Cotton Mills and Factory Acts 1819, was largely ineffective and was superseded over a decade later by the Factory Act 1833 that legislated for two hours of education per day and restricted the hours that children aged between nine and thirteen could work. The amount of time and time of day that a child could work was further restricted by factory legislation introduced in 1844 and 1850. Furthermore, the employment of those under the age of ten was prohibited in all industries by the Factory and Workshop Act of 1878, while in 1901 the minimum age of employment was increased again, this time to twelve years old.

Despite legislation designed to protect the child in the workplace there were no age restrictions or recommended ages for those to be confined in asylums. Beyond the legal definitions associated with child labour a plethora of variables such as place of birth, gender, social standing, parental occupations, and level of education all impacted on the boundaries that one might draw in defining childhood. In fact the age when childhood ended was an issue debated contemporaneously. A Royal Commission appointed in 1819 to investigate the employment of children in the cotton industry stated:

> In general at about the fourteenth year young persons are no longer treated as children; they are not usually chastised by corporal punishment, and at the same time an important change takes place in what may be termed their domestic condition. For the most part they cease to be under the complete control of their parents and guardians. They begin to retain part of their wages. They frequently pay for their own lodging, board and clothing. They usually make their own contracts, and are, in the proper sense of the words, free agents.[3]

For those shaping the first legislation in England and Wales restricting the working hours and conditions of children, the age of fourteen was a turning point. Those that had reached this milestone were effectively 'free agents' in an adult world. Their opinions were not, however, formed with the sole interests of children in mind. In the cotton industries of England, the young provided a reliable, yet inexpensive, workforce. This convenient labour was sourced primarily from amongst destitute children and they were legally bound into employment through the process of Poor Law apprenticeship. The parish apprentice offered the advantage (to employers) of being unpaid and easily replaced if injury, death, or the completion of their term occurred. Katrina Honeyman observed that an apprentice taken on at the age of eight or nine could have potentially worked without pay for up to a dozen years.[4] Consequently, with the advent of factories, apprentices became central to the production process and were an essential element in the industrial labour force. In these circumstances eight or nine was more than a suitable age for a child to enter the world of employment.

Remaining with the Poor Law, the workhouse was another important institution that defined children, both in terms of age and social status. The Poor Law Amendment Act 1834 introduced stricter regulation of welfare and established the 'less eligibility' workhouse as the centrepiece of welfare provision in England and Wales. The effectiveness of this legislation is a discussion for elsewhere, but in 1836 the Poor Law Commission issued a directive that classified paupers in order to segregate them inside workhouses. Boys over thirteen years old were confined with able-bodied men and girls aged sixteen and over were confined with able-bodied women. Clearly, for the Poor Law Commission, the age of childhood was gender specific with their judgements influenced by the presence of unchaste women and prostitutes that might contaminate the moral values of 'innocent' young girls. Poor Law age regulations were revised further in 1838 when the age of fifteen was considered suitable for both boys and girls to enter the adult areas of the workhouse. However, the extent to which these directives were applied has been question by Frank Crompton who suggested that segregation, according to the 1838 guidelines, was not adopted by all Poor Law unions.[5] The enforcement of directives was thus reliant on the enthusiasm of localities and that the lines demarcating childhood remained unclear.

During the nineteenth century the Poor Law was not the sole institutional provider for the young. The Elementary Education Act 1870 recommended school attendance for children aged between five and twelve years old. However, attendance was not compulsory until 1880 and then only for those aged under ten years old. Even after compulsion was introduced, non-attendance remained common and symbolised working-class refusal to accept state-led definitions of childhood.[6] Hugh Cunningham has noted that in 1889 London alone issued 13,000 summonses for the offence of non-attendance at school.[7] It was not until 1918 that the age of compulsory attendance was raised to fourteen, although there had been increases to eleven in 1893 and twelve in 1899. By the turn of the century, the age of thirteen, rather than fourteen, was suitable for entering into employment.

In a privately funded medical sphere there were specialist institutions established that dealt with the needs of the mentally disabled, rather than the mentally ill—the distinction between these medical categories is discussed below. These idiot asylums, as they were called, catered for congenital patients. They have attracted interest from scholars and it is worthwhile exploring the ages for childhood that have been used elsewhere in the historiography. David Wright applied the upper age limit of eighteen in his book on the Royal Earlswood Asylum for Idiots, although he observed that the average age of entry was between nine and eleven.[8] In his study of the Western Counties Idiot Asylum, David Gladstone employed the age limit of fifteen to define those that entered the institution as children.[9] It can be argued that in these institutions the onset of adulthood might have occurred later than it would have done for families of the working poor and destitute whose children were confined in pauper lunatic asylums. During the nineteenth century a period of adolescence came to separate childhood and adult life. Middle-class families were particularly affected because of extended periods of education, apprenticeships, and a trend towards later marriage.[10] Even though the Earlswood and Western Counties idiot asylums received large numbers of the 'respectable' poor they operated according to the bourgeois ideals of their subscribers and were embedded with their own concepts of when childhood ended. Medical institutions more broadly were beginning to define the parameters for children and childhood in the mid-nineteenth century. Subscriber hospitals became common during the period but they excluded children aged under seven from treatment because their high mortality rates were bad for business. Child specific hospitals, such as that on Great Ormond Street in London, were established from the 1850s but they developed much later than similar institutions in Europe that were founded half a century before. These advances in the medical world reflected a changing social and cultural outlook towards protecting the lives of the young.

Detailed historical research has further enhanced ideas of childhood and when this phase of life ended in the past. Keith Snell has demonstrated that the average age for leaving home between the years 1700–1860 was 14.5 years for males and 15.5 years for females in the agricultural sector and 14.3 years for males and 13.5 for females for those apprenticed.[11] Here we can see that the age of fourteen, or thereabouts, was commonly seen as a time for children to leave the family home and be considered as adults. Towards the end of the nineteenth century, the influential child reform campaigner Margaret McMillan argued that the tension between the 'labouring' child and the 'schooled' child needed to be resolved before youngsters of the lower classes could experience healthy growth and improved mental development.[12] Although largely implicit, the age of schooling was used in these instances to define the child. Similarly, scholarship such as that of Harry Hendrick has noted an increased medical concern for children working half or full time, but this again is embedded in the school environment.[13] Moreover, Hilary Marland and Marijke Giswijt-Hofstra have identified and acknowledged the difficulties in defining the child in a health setting at the turn of the twentieth century and ultimately opted for the age of schooling (four to fourteen) as adequate parameters.[14]

Outside of the school, modern scholars have imposed their own ideas of when childhood ended for Victorian and Edwardian youngsters. For example, Ginger Frost adopted the age of fourteen when exploring Victorian childhoods;[15] in their study of the pauper lunatic asylum in

Devon, Melling et al. included the records of those aged up to fifteen;[16] and Kate Gingell applied the age of fourteen in her work on the Powick asylum.[17] Furthermore, Eileen Wallace went up to the age of seventeen when examining child labour in Hertfordshire and Hugh Cunningham in his far-reaching work used the upper age limit of fifteen to define the child.[18] It is evident from the historiography that concepts of childhood were inextricably linked with the fluid and broader contemporary issues of welfare, education, medical and physical hygiene, and the roles of families, the state and medical professionals. Consequently, with the emergence of the eugenics movement towards the end of the nineteenth century, childhood health became intertwined with ideas of race, empire, and national efficiency. Indeed, the impact of these 'scientific' ideas on concepts of childhood are something that we move to shortly.

Thus the parameters for defining a child in the nineteenth century are complex. Nevertheless, a meaningful age boundary has to be applied in order to conduct a worthwhile and significant investigation into the nature and experiences of child insanity. Moving forward the records of those under the age of fourteen at admission to the asylum will be used to conduct the analysis. While this might seem young by modern standards the reasons for such a restriction are grounded in the nineteenth-century context. Royal Commissions, workhouse segregation, apprenticeships, schooling, and labour legislation all indicate that fourteen was viewed as an age for working. Furthermore, in the admission documentation of pauper lunatic asylums those aged fourteen often have an occupation recorded, whereas younger individuals are attributed their parent's occupation such as 'the son of a labourer' or 'daughter of seamstress'.

Five Pauper Lunatic Asylums

Having broadly identified the children under examination and establishing a crucial age parameter for them, it is equally important to turn attention to the environment of the pauper lunatic asylum. Despite the wealth of literature dealing with asylums we know surprisingly little about the majority of institutions. There are of course some exceptions such as The York Retreat, Bethlem, Devon County Asylum, and the Norfolk Asylum.[19] However, to better understand how they functioned, further knowledge of more institutions and a good understanding of the people and experiences of those confined need to be developed. Furthermore, the historical literature has not yet effectively examined how asylums operated in relation to each other and whether they offered a standardised network of care. Considering these lacunae this book has a number of objectives: (i) to understand the experiences and nature of confinement for children admitted to pauper lunatic asylums; (ii) through the prism of children, compare and evaluate the function and purposes of asylums at local, regional, and national levels; (iii) to identify the broad economy of makeshifts, hitherto only partially uncovered, for the treatment of children with mental health problems; (iv) to demonstrate that child insanity was an important social issue of the time. These will be achieved through a comparative analysis of five pauper lunatic asylums. These institutions—Prestwich Asylum in Manchester, Winson Green Asylum in Birmingham, Berrywood Asylum in Northamptonshire, Three Counties Asylum serving Bedfordshire, Hertfordshire, and Huntingdonshire, and Colney Hatch in Middlesex can be placed on an imaginary line from the north-west to the south-east of England, as seen in Fig. 1.1.

By focusing on five asylums a broad and specific illustration of how child insanity was managed during the period can be constructed. Each asylum possessed certain characteristics that make its inclusion important to developing a more complete understanding of the provision offered for children in any network of care. It is also important to note that none of the asylums, or the Medical Superintendents responsible for their operation, took a particularly keen interest in or professed to have a specialism in dealing with child mental illness or disability. This was not always the case and Dr William Parsey at the Warwickshire County Asylum, for instance, established in 1871 a separate idiot institution at the asylum that was geared towards the training of 200 mentally disabled children from the surrounding area.[20] However, this was an exception in the public asylum network and prominent physicians in the field of childhood mental disability such as George Shuttleworth, George Grabham, and John Langdon Down all occupied Medical Superintendent posts at privately funded idiot institutions.[21]

Although more detail about each institution will emerge as we progress, a brief history and description of each is useful at the outset. Beginning with the asylum at Colney Hatch, near Barnet in north London, it was opened on 17 July 1851 and was the second pauper lunatic asylum in the county of Middlesex. Due to its proximity to the metropolis it received a large, heterogeneous population. When the first patients entered it was the biggest and most modern lunatic institution in Europe, catering for 1250 patients initially and at its peak housing in the region of 3500 patients.

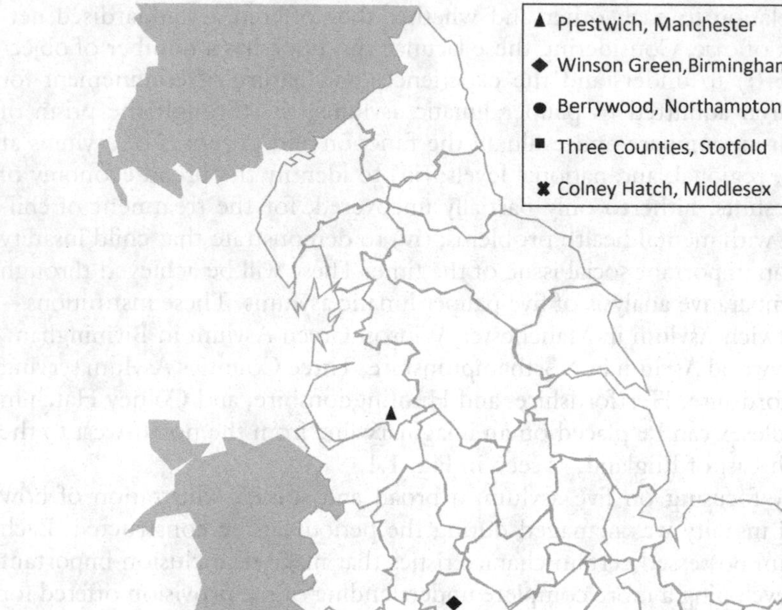

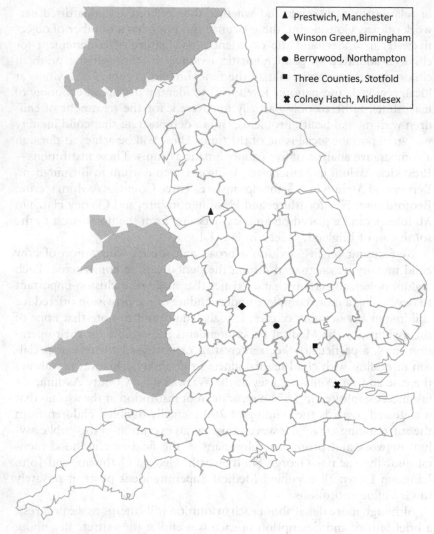

Fig. 1.1 Map of England showing the five asylums

It is included in here because of its size, prominence, and proximity to London.[22]

The Birmingham Borough or Winson Green Asylum, later known as All Saints Hospital, was built in the Winson Green area of the city close to the union workhouse and the prison. Its doors opened to patients in June 1850 when it catered to 300 pauper lunatic patients. By the end of the period, this figure had risen to somewhere in the region of 1200. The asylum at Birmingham is the only borough asylum that features, with the other four all being county asylums. It was designed to serve the city and had a catchment area of three heavily populated and industrial Poor Law unions (Aston, Birmingham, and Kings Heath).

The Prestwich Asylum opened near Manchester on 1 January 1851. It was one of four asylums that provided provision for pauper lunatics in one of Britain's largest and most populous counties, Lancashire; with the others located at Lancaster (1816), Rainhill (1851), and Whittingham (1873). Initially the asylum was built to hold 350 patients but by 1889 it had rapidly expanded to house 2300 pauper lunatics and by 1903 was home to 3135. The asylum was established to provide lunacy provision for the large urban centres of Manchester and Salford, but from 1891 it was administered by the Lancashire Asylums Board (LAB) and began to see more patients from across the county admitted when space was available. At this point in time Lancashire was the global supplier of cotton and the cities of Manchester and Liverpool grew around this trade, employing numerous spinners, weavers, bleachers, and dyers. Outside of the cities there were large cotton mill towns such as Blackburn, Bolton, Burnley, Oldham, and Rochdale. The county, however, was diverse and beyond urban areas there were also significant agricultural spaces meaning that the asylum witnessed admissions from a multitude of backgrounds. Lancashire also experienced considerable migration from Ireland in the post famine years adding to the heterogeneity of the county and its asylum population.[23]

In contrast to the three asylums already mentioned, the Three Counties Asylum, opened on 8 March 1860, and the Northamptonshire Asylum, opened at Berrywood on 30 June 1876, were both in predominantly rural counties.[24] At its opening the Three Counties Asylum had room for 466 patients but by 1894 had expanded to accommodate 1000. The Northamptonshire institution was built to confine 115 patients yet by 1889 it contained over 850 pauper lunatics. In contrast to the institutions in London, Manchester, and Birmingham, these asylums were located in rural areas without dense industry or significant urban populations.[25] Over the period in question, however, they witnessed population shifts to towns. A theme highlighted by Elizabeth Hurren who has demonstrated that in Northamptonshire families traditionally worked the land, but supplemented their incomes with work in the boot and shoe trade, an industry that became much more important by the turn of the twentieth century.[26] The asylums in rural regions have to be considered in a wider context of industrial and urban change. By examining five very different institutions it is possible to conduct a detailed overview of provision for children certified as insane and to also contrast the management of insane populations across geographic regions.

The asylums have left behind an extensive array of records and the children admitted to them have been identified through an examination of admission registers, patient indexes, and patient casebooks. This was a laborious task that gleaned the names, ages, diagnoses, and admission numbers of children but produced limited further detail. The personal stories and experiences of individual children were revealed by using admission numbers to locate their unique casefiles. These recorded the asylum experience of each person admitted to the institution and provide a glimpse into their world. Through this process of research there have been 773 children aged under fourteen identified across the five institutions between the years 1845–1907. This book accounts for these children both quantitatively and qualitatively to gain a better understanding of their experiences living with mental disorder and to comprehend how they moved through systems of welfare and medicine.

Historians and the 'Insane'

To get to the heart of the reasons why children came to be confined in asylums it is important to explore the varied ideas about what it meant to be insane in the nineteenth century. Most, if not all, historical investigations take Michel Foucault's *Histoire de la Folie* as a starting point. In this influential work it was argued that asylums functioned to control deviant elements in communities that had failed or refused to adapt to the needs of emerging industrial society.[27] Foucault contended that from the mid-seventeenth century onwards there was 'a great confinement' of those that affronted bourgeois capitalist sensibilities. These people were not just the mad, but everyone considered to be different from the 'norm' such as beggars, prostitutes, criminals, the disabled, and the elderly. They were lumped together without any medical rationale, primarily because they were considered idle and a drain on resources.

While undoubtedly compelling, Foucault's argument has been criticised for being vague and overly reliant on the French experience during the seventeenth century.[28] Amongst others, Roy Porter has critiqued the chronology of a European-wide 'great confinement' of the insane from 1660 pointing out that the analysis 'falls down' within the English context. State legislation dealing with the insane did not occur in England until 1808 and compulsory asylums did not become law until 1845, almost two centuries after the supposed 'great confinement'.[29] Clearly our understanding of who the insane were, how they were defined, and the function of asylums requires a greater degree of nuance. A more detailed picture has been offered by Andrew Scull, although deviancy still featured heavily.[30] Scull saw asylums as the vehicle that alienists (doctors of the insane) used to claim professional and medical authority over those that had not adapted to capitalist society. However, their efforts were tethered by the admission of long-stay incurable patients that led Scull to conclude that the asylum's 'primary value to the community was as a handy place to which to consign the awkward and unwanted, the useless and potentially troublesome'.[31] This approach recognises that the characteristics, behaviours, and responses to the insane were to some degree a reflection of contemporary social attitudes, but it is still very much an argument that pigeon-holes them as burdensome or unwanted.

More recent scholarship has challenged the notion that the insane were merely society's rejects. Cathy Smith has presented a number of social roles that the asylum fulfilled in order to better understand its occupants. They acted as custodians of dangerous lunatics, a place where the demented or disturbed could be removed from society, a hospice for a range of medical conditions, and a place for drunks to sober up.[32] Smith demonstrated that in the Northampton General Asylum the length of residence was on average between six months and a year. If the asylum was an institution for the confinement of social undesirables the duration of stay did not reflect this.[33] Furthermore, Adair et al. have claimed that in south-west England the workhouse and officials of the Poor Law union, rather than families, played the key role in deciding what type of individuals were sent to the county asylum. Dealing a blow to the suggestion that it was families that sought to deposit unwanted or economically useless members in the asylum.[34]

A foundation of the social control argument has been that asylums predominantly confined the idle and welfare and social reintegration of the individual, unproductive. Peter Bartlett has demonstrated, however, that employment inside the asylums was the 'cornerstone' of bringing about cure and an aid to reintegrating lunatics back into society.[35] Consequently, the asylum was not just a place for the residuum but it was also a crutch for the 'respectable' poor in times of need. Often the institution helped to find employment for recovered lunatics before discharge and the standard of destitution upon entry was rarely enforced. Bartlett even highlights that some asylums provided employment for former patients when they encountered temporary periods of joblessness.[36] The image of asylums as institutions of reform and rehabilitation, working for the welfare and social reintegration of the individual, is asymmetrical to the institution presented by those with a social control perspective. What both schools of thought have in common is that they only focus on adults. By concentrating on children this book helps to provide a more complete understanding of ideas about insanity, the pauper lunatic asylum, and its role in nineteenth-century society.

From historiographical debates it is clear that ideas about insane behaviour were contested and it is therefore appropriate at this point to comment on the language to be used in the rest of the book. Thus far, when children have been mentioned they have been described as 'insane' rather than 'lunatic', 'mentally defective', 'mentally deficient', 'idiotic', or 'imbecile'. These are all terms that were regularly used in medical, welfare, and social situations during the period and they have been used here already in relation to adult patients. To modern ears these might appear vulgar, rude, and offensive but in order to avoid confusing anachronisms they appear as they would in the nineteenth-century context.[37] 'Insane' was a legal term that encompassed the spectrum of mental illnesses and disabilities across the nineteenth century. However, as we progress the distinctions between illnesses and disabilities require a greater degree of clarification. 'Lunacy' was a catch-all term for those with acquired and temporary conditions, but it did not accurately apply to the large number of children found in asylums that had from birth displayed characteristics of mental disability. The diagnoses for these conditions were 'idiocy' and 'imbecility' and their definitions feature in the next chapter. The distinctions have been acknowledged in the historiography and the last two decades have seen important contributions examining the historical experiences of mental disability from the early modern period through to the twentieth century.[38]

Throughout the nineteenth century it is vital to keep in mind that concepts of insanity and the insane were evolving. Part of this process was the introduction and acceptance of other labels for mental disorder, such as 'mentally defective', 'weak-minded', and 'feeble-minded' that had their roots outside of medical discourse. These terms were the product of an intellectual framework heavily influenced by social Darwinism and the nascent eugenic movement. The concept of mental deficiency developed as a sub-category for those considered not mentally disabled but also not of 'normal' intellect. Janet Saunders has examined campaigns in the 1860s and 1870s to quarantine mentally deficient individuals with criminal tendencies.[39] She has suggested that the theory of 'progressive degeneration', elaborated in France in 1857 and brought to the British context by Henry Maudsley, was vital to the arguments of those campaigning for segregation. A forerunner to the eugenics movement, the idea of degeneration suggested that there were inherited defects in the weak minded, and that mental deficiency and criminality were different points on the same slope to idiocy.[40] The march towards quarantine, however, eventually faltered when prison medical superintendents questioned the validity of degeneration arguments.[41]

In the years following these campaigns, Mathew Thomson has argued that mental deficiency became a specific and widespread problem as a consequence of the introduction of elementary education in 1870 and with it increased attention to the intellectual abilities of children. In parallel to these educative reforms, a downturn in the British economy made it more difficult for the mentally deficient to find employment opportunities and support themselves in the wider community. Eugenics was an important factor that raised fears about national degeneration and the susceptibility of the poor to mental weakness at a time when the mentally deficient appeared to become more ubiquitous in a community setting. However, Thomson suggests that at this point in time eugenic influence was not always paramount and humanitarian ideas about helping the incapable held equal weight.[42]

A specific exploration of attitudes towards the mentally deficient during this period is provided by Mark Jackson who examines the contribution of the campaigner Mary Dendy and her Sandlebridge Special School founded in north-west England in 1902.[43] She was specifically concerned with the feeble-minded, a group that like the weak-minded, occupied a 'borderland' between what might be considered 'normal' mental abilities and idiocy. Jackson highlights that this group were thought a threat to national decline because of their propensity for 'criminality, bestiality, promiscuity, and excessive fertility'.[44] Dendy campaigned for the permanent segregation of this class of 'defectives' in order to preserve the social order. By the turn of the twentieth century, Jackson argues that attitudes towards reforming and improving those with mental disabilities had been overtaken by constructions of them as pathologically distinct and different from ordinary society. His use of photographs demonstrated that 'medical writers not only agreed that mental defectives presented a variety of characteristic (and supposedly objective) physical abnormalities that could be used in diagnosis but also that those abnormalities could be accurately portrayed in photographs'.[45] The use of visual images reinforced ideas about the feeble-minded and galvanised medical professionals who could identify such individuals to protect society from their supposed threat.

The children confined inside pauper lunatic asylums have received limited attention from historians. To date the most thorough overview is that conducted by Melling et al. in their examination of the Devon County Asylum. Their approach explores the reasons for admission to the asylum and the importance of family and community interactions in the process of certification. Individual experiences of the children are overlooked but the Devon analysis still provides a useful starting point. Significantly, Melling et al. concluded that the active co-operation of family members in the process of admitting a lunatic child was vital. With the most effective way of securing admission being to present the child, no matter how small, as a threat to the family environment.[46] In this instance admission notes and Certificates of Insanity are examined as complex transactions between agents with differing motives. Melling et al. argue that the physicians responsible for admission were striving to demonstrate their own professional expertise while simultaneously attempting to translate witness statements from family and lay quarters into coherent legal documents; all of this while abiding by the strategies and requirements of the institution. Consequently, the children admitted to the asylum were administrative, legal and social constructions rather than medical or therapeutic ones.[47] The Devon study covers the years 1845–1914 and discovered a modest number of children admitted to the asylum. Correctly, it acknowledged that the majority of insane children remained outside the walls of the asylum, being treated either domestically or in workhouse provision. The failure to admit children was, in their opinion, a reflection of the unwillingness by professionals and administrators to deal with child insanity in the same manner as insanity among adults. Subsequently, the argument is grounded in the context of wider campaigning and legislative action for a specific provision for children.[48] The broad reasons for admission revolved around the danger or disruption the child posed in domestic or workhouse care. Threats to younger siblings or to the smooth operation of the workhouse were viewed as important justifications for confining a child within the asylum. Inside of workhouses Melling et al. highlight the strained relationship between Medical Officers that often sought to remove troublesome children and Poor Law Guardians that wanted them retained in the workhouse, mainly for financial reasons.[49] Through this analytical lens the deviant and destructive child found their way to the asylum, while the more placid was retained and made useful through work.

Despite its value, there are a number of shortcomings in the analysis of the Devon asylum. Firstly, the isolated and insular approach to a single rural institutional experience is problematic; it is unclear how far any conclusions can be extrapolated to a national level. Secondly, the research provides only a limited discussion of the impact of non-lunacy legislation and social movements on children's lives, such as the introduction of regulations tackling education and employment, the emergence of Evangelical reformers, and the impact of eugenic ideas. Where non-lunacy legislation is examined the analysis is brief and from a top-down perspective. Finally, the constructions of child insanity are too narrow. Discussions of conditions such as epilepsy lack depth and are dismissed due to the frequency with which they occurred in the Devon experience. On occasion the authors are unconcerned with the medical circumstances of those admitted; the prevalence of adolescent males in their cohort is explained by stating that 'the "problem" of the child lunatic was more particularly an issue of how the behaviour of older children and adolescents was to be managed'.[50] This judgement lacks analytical rigour and often the ailments of child patients are accepted within the boundaries of the insane adult population. In their defence the investigation undertaken by Melling et al. was not intended to be a comprehensive discussion of child insanity in England; however, it does generate a number of important issues, such as the 'types' of children admitted, the nature of their conditions, and how they were managed in asylums, that need to be explored.

The perception of child insanity as a wider social issue has been addressed by Amy Rebok Rosenthal, who demonstrates the concern of alienists and leading philanthropists for children and families that did not conform to acceptable social norms.[51] This overview is a 'top–down' examination of concerns about insanity during the period. Rosenthal does not acknowledge the role of the family and children in the process of confinement and sees asylums as custodial institutions. Any potential agency of families is overlooked and the asylum is not considered as part of a broader range of welfare possibilities accessible to the poor. Rosenthal provides a thorough technical overview of broad attitudes towards insane children from the authorities and prominent alienists, but her analysis is not furnished with an adequate discussion of the East Kent County Asylum that she focuses on. For example, while there are a handful of emblematic case studies presented, Rosenthal does not state how many children were admitted to the institutions, the diagnoses from which they suffered, or how they departed the asylum. These are key elements that will be addressed here to broaden our understanding of insane children in this institution during the period.

The experience of mental debility rather than institutional confinement has been presented in David Wright's study of the Royal Earlswood Idiot Asylum.[52] The children admitted to this institution were not of the pauper class and they were all diagnosed as being mentally disabled. Nevertheless this work is important as it highlights and explores the central role of family in diagnosis and securing the necessary subscriber recommendations for admission. Wright observes that while most historical work focuses on the generic lunatic, the more specific afflictions of idiocy and imbecility have been neglected. Those confined at Earlswood were chronic patients suffering from a mental disability. Because they could not be cured, it is thought that pauper lunatic asylums were unenthusiastic about their admission and they were left to fester in workhouse lunatic wards unless they became violent or disruptive.[53] A key distinction between Earlswood and pauper asylums is that a time limit of five years of confinement was placed upon patients to prevent the 'silting up' of the institution with the chronically disabled. Furthermore, Wright provides a detailed survey of the specific medical provision and training that was available for idiot children at Earlswood, a provision often absent from the care available in county asylums.

The treatment of insane children confined within the poor law union workhouse has received even less attention than those in asylums. In his book, *Workhouse Children*, Frank Crompton provides a limited discussion of the children maintained in the Worcestershire workhouses.[54] Unfortunately, he is largely unconcerned with issues surrounding the confinement of insane children and chooses to focus on an administrative overview of lunacy legislation and its application within the workhouse to draw some general conclusions on how it impacted child lunatics. The main point arising from Crompton's investigation is that insane children were regularly kept within the children's ward of the workhouse on the condition that they were not disruptive. He has also noted that in Worcestershire the Poor Law Guardians were tempted to avoid labelling children as dangerous in order to avoid incurring the increased costs of asylum care.[55] Any empirical discussion of the number of insane children confined within the workhouse or for departures from the workhouse to the county asylum once it opened in 1852 is not included. By extending the focus to wider avenues of care, it will be possible to garner a greater knowledge of how differing institutions, such as the workhouse, managed children with mental impairment.

Thus it can be seen that the literature regarding child lunacy and the provision for insane children is at best patchy.[56] In the pages that follow a comprehensive and comparative analysis of child insanity and the provisions in place to deal with it will be conducted. While some of the analysis resonates with that of Melling et al. and Wright it will also deviate significantly. Chapter 2 explores the various constructions of child insanity and takes an in-depth look at how mental disability evolved and was diagnosed during this period. Furthermore, it offers a detailed discussion of the process and administration of admission while exploring elements of childhood experience inside the asylum. Chapter 3 continues to focus on children in the asylum, but looks more specifically at how the five asylums operated in relation, if at all, to each other. It observes a number of similarities and differences across the regions and argues that typology was more important than regionality in the function of any asylum 'network'. Chapter 4 marks a shift and begins to 'look out' from the asylum to a wider economy of medical care that existed during the period. It places the asylum in this network of broader relief and assesses its role in relation to other institutions operating at the time. Chapter 5 moves beyond the asylum and investigates both private and public spaces used to manage insane children. It considers increased state regulation in education and child welfare alongside philanthropic efforts to emphasise the broader social importance of child mental health between the years 1845–1907. The final chapter offers conclusions as to the nature, experience and significance of child insanity and argues that the findings of this book have an importance stretching beyond the histories of childhood and insanity.

Notes

1. C. Heywood, 'Children's Work in Countryside and City,' in Paula Fass (ed.), *The Routledge History of Childhood in the Western World* (London: Routledge, 2013), 125–141.
2. V. Zelizer, *Pricing the Priceless Child: The Changing Social Value of Children* (New York: Princeton University Press, 1985).
3. Cited in H. Cunningham, *Children and Childhood in Western Society since 1500* (London: Longman 1995), p. 140.
4. K. Honeyman, *Child Workers in England, 1780–1820: Parish Apprentices and the Making of the Early Industrial Labour Force* (Aldershot: Ashgate, 2007), p. 7.
5. F. Crompton, *Workhouse Children* (Stroud: Sutton, 1997), p. 38.
6. A. Digby and P. Searby, *Children, School and Society in Nineteenth-Century England* (London: Macmillan, 1981), p. 13.
7. Cunningham, *Children and Childhood*, pp. 103–106.
8. D. Wright, *Mental Disability in Victorian England: The Earlswood Asylum, 1847–1901* (Oxford: Clarendon, 2001).
9. D. Gladstone, 'The Changing Dynamic of Institutional Care: The Western Counties Idiot Asylum, 1864–1914,' in D. Wright and A. Digby (eds.), *From Idiocy to Mental Deficiency, Historical Perspectives on People with Learning Disabilities* (London: Routledge 1996), pp. 134–160, p. 142.
10. R. P. Neuman, 'Masturbation, Madness and the Modern Concepts of Childhood and Adolescence,' *Journal of Social History*, 8/3 (1975), pp. 1–27.
11. K. D. M. Snell, *Annals of the Labouring Poor: Social Change and Agrarian England, 1660–1900* (Cambridge: Cambridge University Press, 1985), p. 326.
12. C. Steedman, 'Bodies, Figures and Physiology: Margaret McMillan and the Late Nineteenth-Century Remaking of Working-Class Childhood,' in R. Cooter (ed.), *In the Name of the Child: Health and Welfare, 1880–1940* (London: Routledge, 1992), pp. 19–44, pp. 21–26.
13. H. Hendrick, 'Child Labour, Medical Capital, and the School Medical Service, c.1890–1918,' in Cooter (ed.), *In the Name of the Child*, pp. 45–71.
14. H. Marland and M. Gijswijt-Hofstra, 'Cultures of Child Health in Britain and the Netherlands in the Twentieth Century,' in Marland and Gijswijt-Hofstra (eds.), *Cultures of Child Health in Britain and the Netherlands in the Twentieth Century* (Amsterdam: Editions Rodopi, 2003), pp. 7–30, p. 8.
15. G. Frost, *Victorian Childhoods* (London: ABC, 2008), p. 4.

16. J. Melling, R. Adair, and B. Forsythe, '"A Proper Lunatic for Two Years": Pauper Lunatic Children in Victorian and Edwardian England. Child Admissions to the Devon County Lunatic Asylum, 1845–1914,' *Journal of Social History*, 31/2 (1997), pp. 371–405, p. 374.
17. K. Gingell, 'The Forgotten Children: Children Admitted to a County Asylum between 1854–1900,' *The Psychiatrist*, 25/11 (2001), p. 432.
18. E. Wallace, *Children of the Labouring Poor: The Working Lives of Children in Nineteenth-Century* Hertfordshire (Hatfield: Hertfordshire Publications, 2010), p. 5; Cunningham, *Children and Childhood*, p. 17.
19. For the York Retreat see A. Digby, 'The Changing Profile of a Nineteenth Century Asylum: The York Retreat,' *Psychological Medicine*, 14/4 (1984), pp. 739–748; Digby, *Madness, Morality and Medicine: A Study of the York Retreat* (Cambridge: Cambridge University Press, 1985); Digby, 'Moral Treatment at the Retreat, 1796–1846,' in W.F. Bynum, R. Porter, and M. Shepherd (eds.), *The Anatomy of Madness: Essays in the History of Psychiatry*, vol. 2, pp. 52–72; L. Wannell, 'Patients' Relatives and Psychiatric Doctors: Letter Writing in the York Retreat, 1875–1910,' *Social History of Medicine*, 20/2 (2007), pp. 297–313; for Bethlem see C. Arnold, *Bedlam: London and Its* Mad (London: Pocket, 2008); A. Scull, C. MacKenzie, and N. Hervey, *Masters of Bedlam: The Transformation of the Mad-Doctoring Trade* (New Jersey: Princeton University Press, 1996); for Devon see J. Melling et al., 'A Proper Lunatic'; B. Forsythe, J. Melling, and R. Adair, 'The New Poor Law and the County Pauper Lunatic Asylum—The Devon Experience 1834–1884,' *Social History of Medicine*, 9/3 (1996), pp. 335–355; Adair, Melling, and Forsythe, 'Migration, Family Structure and Pauper Lunacy in Victorian England: Admissions to the Devon County Pauper Lunatic Asylum, 1845–1900,' *Continuity and Change*, 12/3 (1997), pp. 373–401; Adair, Forsythe, and Melling, 'A Danger to the Public? Disposing of Pauper Lunatics in Late-Victorian and Edwardian England: Plympton St Mary Union and the Devon County Asylum, 1867–1914,' *Medical History*, 42/1 (1998), pp. 1–25; for Norfolk see S. Cherry, *Mental Health Care in Modern England: The Norfolk Lunatic Asylum/St. Andrews Hospital* (Woodbridge: Boydell, 2003).
20. M. Archer, *Idiocy and Institutionalisation in Late Victorian Britain. The Warwick County Idiot Asylum 1852 to 1877* (University of Warwick: Unpublished MA Thesis 2010).
21. D. Wright, *Downs: The History of a Learning Disability* (Oxford: Oxford University Press, 2011).
22. R. Hunter and I. MacAlpine, *Psychiatry for the Poor: 1851 Colney Hatch Asylum—Friern Hospital 1973: A Medical and Social History* (London: Dawsons, 1974).

23. C. Cox, H. Marland, and S. York, 'Emaciated, Exhausted, and Excited: The Bodies and Minds of the Irish in Late Nineteenth-Century Lancashire Asylums,' *Journal of Social History*, 46/2 (2012), pp. 500–524; Cox, Marland, and York, 'Itineraries and Experiences of Insanity: Irish Migration and the Management of Mental Illness in Nineteenth-Century Lancashire,' in Cox and Marland (eds.), *Migration, Health and Ethnicity in the Modern World* (Basingstoke: Palgrave Macmillan, 2013), pp. 36–60; Cox and Marland, '"A Burden on the County": Madness, Institutions of Confinement and the Irish Patient in Victorian Lancashire,' *Social History of Medicine*, 28/2 (2015), pp. 263–287.
24. An explanation for the late establishment of the Northamptonshire asylum is provided by C. Smith, 'Parsimony, Power, and Prescriptive Legislation: The Politics of Pauper Lunacy in Northamptonshire, 1845–1876,' *Bulletin of the History of Medicine*, 81/2 (2007), pp. 359–385.
25. These regional characteristics were identified at the time by the prominent alienists J. Bucknill and D. Tuke and expressed in: *A Manual of Psychological Medicine: Containing the History, Nosology, Description, Statistics, Diagnosis, Pathology and Treatment of Insanity* (London: John Churchill, 1858).
26. E. Hurren, *Protesting About Pauperism: Poverty, Politics and Poor Relief in Late-Victorian England, 1870–1900* (Woodbridge: Boydell & Brewer, 2008).
27. M. Foucault, *Madness and Civilisation: A History of Insanity in the Age of Reason* (London: Routledge, reprint 2001) originally *Histoire de la folie á l'age classique* (1961).
28. R. Porter, *Mind-Forg'd Manacles: A History of Madness in England from Restoration to Regency* (London: Athlone, 1987), pp. 110–112; a further critique of Foucault is provided by P. Spierenburg, "The Sociogenesis of Confinement and its Development in Early Modern Europe,' in P. Spierenburg (ed.), *Emergence of Carceral Institution: Prisons, Galleys and Lunatic Asylums* (Rotterdam: Centrum Voor Maatscappij Geschiedenis, Erasmus Universiteit, 1984), pp. 9–77.
29. R. Porter, *Mind-Forg'd Manacles*, p. 111.
30. A. Scull, *Museums of Madness: The Social Organization of Insanity in Nineteenth-Century England* (London: Allen Lane, 1979), p. 612; see also A. Scull, *The Most Solitary of Afflictions: Madness and Society in Britain 1700–1900* (London: Yale University Press, 1993).
31. A. Scull, *Museums of Madness*, p. 612.
32. C. Smith, 'Family, Community and the Victorian Asylum: A Case Study of Northampton General Lunatic Asylum and its Pauper Lunatics,' *Family and Community History*, 9/2 (2006), pp. 109–124, p. 119; also see Wright, 'Getting Out of the Asylum: Understanding the Confinement of

the Insane in the Nineteenth Century,' *Social History of Medicine*, 10/1 (1997), pp. 137–155.

33. Ibid., Smith, p. 111.
34. R. Adair, B. Forsythe, and J. Melling, 'A Danger to the Public? Disposing of Pauper Lunatics in Late Victorian and Edwardian England: Plympton St. Mary Union and the Devon County Asylum, 1867–1914,' *Medical History*, 42/1 (1998), pp. 1–25.
35. P. Bartlett, 'The Asylum and the Poor Law: The Productive Alliance,' in J. Melling (ed.), *Insanity, Institutions and Society, 1800–1914* (London: Routledge, 1999), pp. 48–67, p. 58.
36. Ibid.
37. S. J. Taylor, '"All His Ways are Those of an Idiot": The Admission, Treatment of and Social Reaction to Two 'Idiot' Children of the Northampton Pauper Lunatic Asylum, 1877–1883,' *Family and Community History*, 15/1 (2012), pp. 34–43; also Taylor, 'Insanity, Philanthropy and Emigration: Dealing with Insane Children in Late-Nineteenth-Century North-West England,' *History of Psychiatry*, 25/2 (2014), pp. 224–236.
38. Most importantly is the collection of essays included in D. Wright and A. Digby, *From Idiocy to Mental Deficiency*; also: P. Rushton, 'Lunatics and Idiots: Mental Disorder, the Community, and the Poor Law in North East England 1600–1800," *Medical History*, 32/1 (1988), pp. 34–50; Wright, *Earlswood*.
39. J. Saunders, "Quarantining the Weak-Minded: Psychiatric Definitions of Degeneracy and the Late-Victorian Asylum,' in W.F. Bynum, R. Porter, and M. Shepherd (eds.), *The Anatomy of Madness: Essays in the History of Psychiatry*, vol. III (London: Routledge, 1988), pp. 273–296.
40. Ibid., p. 277.
41. Ibid., p. 288.
42. M. Thomson, *The Problem of Mental Deficiency: Eugenics, Democracy, and Social Policy in Britain c.1870–1959* (Oxford: Clarendon, 1998), p. 297.
43. M. Jackson, *The Borderland of Imbecility: Medicine, Society and the Fabrication of the Feeble Mind in late Victorian and Edwardian England* (Manchester: Manchester University Press, 2000).
44. M. Jackson, '"Grown-up Children": Understandings of Health and Mental Deficiency in Edwardian England,' in Giswijt-Hofstra and Marland (eds.), *Cultures of Child Health in Britain and the Netherlands in the Twentieth Century* (Amsterdam: Rodopi, 2003), pp. 149–168, p. 150.
45. M. Jackson, 'Images of Deviance: Visual Representations of Mental Defectives in Early Twentieth-Century Medical Texts,' *The British Journal for the History of Science*, 28/3 (1995), pp. 319–337, p. 337.
46. Melling et al., 'Proper Lunatic'.

47. Ibid., p. 376.
48. Ibid., p. 373.
49. Ibid., p. 383.
50. Melling, 'Proper Lunatic,' p. 376.
51. A. Rebok Rosenthal, "Insanity, Family and Community in Late-Victorian Britain,' in A. Borsay and P. Dale (eds.), *Disabled Children: Contested Caring, 1850–1979* (London: Pickering & Chatto, 2012), pp. 29–42.
52. Wright, *Earlswood*; following the success of the Earlswood Idiot Asylum other institutions were established using the same model in other parts of England. Also see: Gladstone, 'The Changing Dynamic of Institutional Care'.
53. Ibid., p. 21.
54. Crompton, *Workhouse Children*.
55. Ibid., pp. 83–86.
56. While this research deals specifically with lunatic children in England it is also important to mention here that the institutionalisation of children in Scotland has been presented by I. Hutchinson, 'Institutionalization of Mentally Impaired Children in Scotland c.1855–1914,' *History of Psychiatry*, 22/4 (2011), pp. 416–433.

CHAPTER 2

'Much Below Insects, and so Little Above Sensitive Plants': Constructing the Insane Child

On 14 May 1860, Sarah Ann Goodman, a twelve-year-old pauper lunatic, was admitted to the Three Counties Asylum. On her arrival, like all other patients, she was allocated a casefile, a space where observations about her health and condition were recorded while confined. During the process of admission she received no comment on her mental health other than a brief diagnosis of 'idiocy' and general medical observations of her did not commence until 6 August 1878. By this time Sarah Goodman was thirty years old and had been an asylum resident for over eighteen years. Throughout her confinement she received only six further casefile entries, the final one noting that on 2 October 1886 she was 'very feeble, cannot leave her chair without aid'. Somewhat frustratingly, but perhaps fittingly, this glimpse into Goodman's asylum experience related not to her mental well-being but her physical condition, and does not reveal the fate of the individual. She may have seen out the last of her days in the asylum or, and as we will discover more unlikely, she could have left the institution and reintegrated into society. Goodman's case will be returned to later, but her experience, or the failure to record (a detailed) one at least, encapsulates many of the problems facing those that want to delve deeper into the experiences of children living with mental ill-health in England's county asylums.

The narratives, experiences, and diagnoses of childhood mental illness are complex and constructed at a formative time for psychological and psychiatric medicine. A range of social, cultural, and scientific ideas meshed

S.J. Taylor, *Child Insanity in England, 1845-1907*, Palgrave Studies in the History of Childhood, DOI 10.1007/978-1-137-60027-1_2

to provide wide and varied understandings of what it meant to be insane. Furthermore, the majority of children were diagnosed during a turbulent intellectual time when the working poor in general were being viewed through a social Darwinist lens that both categorised and stigmatised them. A certification of insanity was thus more than a medical construction and more a social comment on family life and childhood. By revealing how the mental impairments of children were constructed it is possible to better understand their experiences, how medical provision accommodated them, and what it meant to be a child living with disability at this time.

Administering Pauper Lunacy

The legislation dealing with asylums and the administration of the insane, both children and adults, evolved over the first half of the nineteenth century. Foucault famously declared that a 'great confinement' of deviant populations occurred across Europe from the 1660s. But in England and Wales the first state-funded asylums were not built until after the County Asylums Act 1808, and even then they were not compulsory.[1] Prior to this Act of Parliament a system of for-profit mad-houses and charitable hospitals existed that confined the mad, as well as vagrants, beggars, and the idle.[2] The permissive nature of the Act meant that progress was slow and the legislation was amended in 1815 to encourage counties to borrow funds in order to expedite the process.[3] Success, however, was limited and by 1828, twenty years after the first asylums act, only ten counties, out of a possible fifty-two, had built specialist institutions. These were most commonly provincial, being built in Bedfordshire, Cornwall, Gloucestershire, Lancashire, Lincoln, Norfolk, Nottinghamshire, Staffordshire, Suffolk, and Yorkshire.[4] This growth in the public sector was mirrored by the creation of private asylums in Oxford, Liverpool, Northampton and Staffordshire that were maintained through patient fees and charitable donations. The development of asylums was thus uneven in the years prior to 1845 and far from representative of a state-sponsored campaign to remove deviant elements from society.

The early asylums, although smaller, provided a model for the later county institutions that were erected across the country. They adopted and refined a system of moral therapy/treatment that was adopted in the compulsory system. This was developed initially by Phillipe Pinel, a French Physician, and adopted in England at the York Retreat—a private institution founded by the Tuke family of Quakers in 1796. It was introduced to public asylums in 1839 by John Conolly at Hanwell, the first Middlesex county asylum . In the years immediately before and after 1845 moral treatment was the cornerstone of treatment towards the insane. It did away with the barbaric and cruel practices that had been associated with caring for the mad in the seventeenth and eighteenth centuries and focused on humane and moral methods of bringing about recovery. A core element of this therapeutic concept was the employment of patients in tasks designed to benefit the smooth running of the asylum. As such moral treatment turned asylums into institutions of productivity and improvement, rather than regulation, surveillance, and custody.[5] Whilst this seems a positive shift in approach, at least for those confined, the motives for the change were questioned by Foucault who believed that, rather than being humane, moral treatment was in fact a repressive act. To him the physical shackles of earlier periods were simply replaced with invisible ones that imprisoned the patient through their own guilt and anxiety.[6] Len Smith argues that these techniques aimed at bringing about cure even if they had only limited success.[7] But a curative philosophy, he argues, was evident from the process of committal and in situations where recovery was not possible, the focus switched to the alleviation of symptoms. The practices and treatments that were experienced in these early institutions were vital in shaping the responses to insanity that developed in the compulsory asylum system that emerged later in the century.

The dual legislation of the Lunacy and County Asylums Acts 1845 made it compulsory for counties to provide provision for their pauper insane and to inspect the premises used for this purpose.[8] The centralised inspectorate of the Commissioners in Lunacy, who regulated this provision, was also established by this legislation. They inspected all receptacles of lunatics on an annual basis and ensured that they were in compliance with legislative guidelines. They also enforced rules of the admission process, making sure that all certifications were issued in line with administrative demands. These measures were designed to prevent the wrongful confinement of the sane population.[9] A discussion of this process is vital to understanding how and why children came to be certified as insane and confined inside asylums.

The first stage of certification was the Poor Law Medical Officer. He, the position was always held by a man, had to inform the Parish Officers within three days of having identified a potential pauper lunatic. In turn, a Justice of the Peace (JP) was then notified within three days by the parish, who arranged for the alleged lunatic to be examined with the assistance of a doctor or medical officer. If insanity was confirmed the medical man completed a Certificate of Insanity and the JP issued a Reception Order that dispatched the insane pauper to the county asylum. These legal steps for certifying insanity and admitting an individual to an asylum were all conducted within the bureaucratic machinery of the Poor Law—the asylum was effectively excluded from selecting its own patients.[10]

This teleological process was, however, not always strictly enforced and often exceptions were made. For instance, on 14 February 1863, seven-year-old George Hamilton was sent, rather unconventionally, directly to Colney Hatch Asylum by the Commissioners in Lunacy.[11] He was said to be dangerous and suicidal, but the medical observation conducted on his entry to the asylum stated that 'why [he was sent] is difficult to discover' and the boy was discharged two weeks later after displaying no symptoms of insanity. Hamilton was initially considered dangerous which might help to explain the need for regulation; in comparison, the admission of the non-dangerous, or as they were described harmless, depended on the discretion of the Relieving Officer and JP. The importance of dangerousness was enshrined in law with the 1846 amendment to the Lunacy Act clearly stating that a detention order should only be issued to dangerous persons. This led to large numbers of the harmless insane being maintained in workhouses or outside of the institutions of lunacy—a less expensive solution for the publicly funded Poor Law and technically contravening the law—often to the frustration of doctors resident in the asylum.[12] The official process also implied that the active agents in the admission of lunatics were Medical Officers and JPs. Until relatively recently it had been assumed that the patients themselves and their families held no agency.[13]

As well as creating a process for certifying the insane, the County Asylums Act established a public network of asylums for accommodating pauper lunatics. Vieda Skultans has suggested that 'the moral outrage felt upon the discovery of the revolting and inhumane conditions endured by the insane and partly by the new found faith in the possibility of cure' prompted the development of this provision.[14] The curative ambitions of new asylums were, however, curiously not included in the wording of the 1845 legislation. The Lunacy Act stated 'any lunatic, idiot or person of unsound mind' should be confined, but not necessarily cured—which had the effect of expanding the problem of lunacy to fit the increasing size of the asylum solution in the years following 1845.[15] Moreover, a further observation was that neither the Lunacy Act nor the County Asylums Act legislated for the ages of those that could be certified insane nor did they provide guidelines on age limits for those confined within asylums.[16]

The law was again altered in 1862 when the Lunacy Laws Amendment Act officially allowed the detention of the non-dangerous insane poor in workhouses and in 1867 when the Metropolitan Poor Act permitted the building of Poor Law Asylums for the non-dangerous insane within the metropolitan area. These measures were designed to ease the problem of overcrowding that many asylums suffered and consequently by the 1870s the county asylum was by no means the only institution that catered for the needs of the insane. While these developments marked a shift where the workhouse could legally be utilised as an institution of care for the insane, as well as a punitive measure for the able-bodied poor, they were also particularly important for children who, because of their high mortality rates, often occupied a grey area in the eyes of medical men. The alternative spaces that developed to cater for the insane meant that a broader economy of care existed, especially as understandings of childhood disorders came under more scrutiny.[17]

The increased focus on the mental impairments of children was given legal status by the Idiots Act 1886 which made specific provision for idiots and imbeciles as a separate group from lunatics.[18] It superseded the Lunacy Acts that were 'considered unnecessary where the patients kept are idiots and imbeciles'.[19] Idiots were no longer legally considered the remit of county asylums and section 17 explicitly stated that '"idiots" or "imbeciles" do not include lunatics, "lunatic" does not mean or include idiot or imbecile'.[20] The 1886 Act provided local authorities with the option of building facilities for the education and training of idiots. But like other, earlier, permissive lunacy legislation it was not enthusiastically adopted by localities.[21] To further complicate the situation, and perhaps highlight the limited understanding of mental health issues at this point in time, the distinctions between lunatics and idiots were again muddied, just four years later, with the 1890 Lunacy Act which stated, a '"lunatic" shall be construed to mean any person—*idiot*, lunatic or of unsound mind and incapable of managing himself or his affairs'.[22] Despite the confusion of nomenclature the 1886 Idiots Act ran in parallel to the 1890 Lunacy Act until it was replaced by the Mental Deficiency Act in 1913.

The 1890 Lunacy Act consolidated previous legislation into one Act. It also transferred responsibility for asylums to the recently established county or borough councils and extended the requirement of a JP's orders for private patients.[23] A further key aim was to provide greater protection against illegal or incorrect confinement. Kathleen Jones argues that the Act heavily reflected the weight of the legal minds that created it, suggesting the legislation contained 'every safeguard which could possibly be devised against illegal confinement'.[24] The 1890 Act, whilst vital in a legal sense, only served to continue the misunderstandings surrounding the definitions of differing forms of mental illness.

Constructions of Child Insanity

Reflecting medical understanding of insanity in the mid-Victorian era, the descriptions, symptoms and experiences of mental ill-health, not only amongst children but for adults too, were varied and at times fluid. This meant that asylum populations were large and heterogeneous.[25] Consequently, child insanity cannot be pigeon-holed into one specific model that was representative of all children admitted to asylums. At the same time it is, however, possible to identify distinct characteristics that featured heavily in descriptions of child mental illness and disability. Diagnoses for children, as can be seen by Table 2.1, were wide-ranging. Idiocy and imbecility, the most common, were permanent states of mental disability, most often congenital and with the former being more severe than the latter.[26] Mania was applied to the impulsive and thoughtless, it was a temporary condition that was curable and could be triggered by numerous factors. Similarly, melancholia was a state of depression that could range from being relatively mild to suicidal, it was also considered a temporary condition. Dementia was the decay of the mind and although in our modern understanding it affects mainly older patients there were a small number of children that received this diagnosis. Displaying the liquid nature of insanity at this time, feeble-mindedness emerged as a distinct category later in the period and described those that occupied a perceived grey area between normal intellectual abilities and imbecility. And finally, epilepsy or 'fits', though poorly understand during the period, was not supposed to be treated in asylums—it was considered as both cause and consequence of mental disability and often was listed as a secondary factor.[27]

From Table 2.1 it can be observed that children were most often admitted to asylums suffering with the mental disabilities of idiocy and imbecility and that the temporary mental illnesses of lunacy, such as mania and melancholia, were more commonly found in adult patients. Also, looking at the child patients in more detail it can be seen that in all of the

Table 2.1 Diagnoses for children by asylum and gender

	Birmingham M-F	*Colney Hatch M-F*	*Manchester M-F*	*Northampton M-F*	*Three Counties M-F*	*Total M-F*
Idiocy	20–14	64–15	15–13	119–78	58–39	276–159
Imbecility	9–6	50–23	9–7	11–6	17–12	96–54
Mania	2–6	24–14	7–7	2–2	10–11	45–40
Dementia	0–3	3–1	1–4	0–2	2–0	6–10
Melancholy	1–3	7–1	1–0	1–0	0–0	10–4
Epilepsy	3–0	4–0	1–3	3–0	7–1	18–4
Feeble-minded	0–0	1–2	1–0	2–0	1–3	5–5
Paralysed	0–0	2–0	0–0	2–0	0–0	4–0
Moral insanity	0–0	0–0	1–0	0–0	0–0	1–0
Poverty	0–0	0–0	0–0	0–0	0–1	0–1
Not insane	0–0	2–0	1–0	0–0	1–0	4–0
Not known	20–8	0–0	0–1	0–1	1–0	21–10
Total	55–40	157–56	37–35	140–89	97–67	486–287

Source: BCL, Male Patient Casebooks, MS344/12/2 & 2a, MS344/12/5, MS344/12/7-9, MS344/12/11-14, MS344/12/20-22, MS344/12/27; BCL, Female Patient Casebooks, MS344/12/41-47, MS344/12/49-51, MS344/12/53 & 54, MS344/12/56 & 57, MS344/12/60-63; BCL, Patient Index, MS344/11/1 & 2; LMA, Colney Hatch Male Patient Casebooks, H12/CH/B/13/001-61; LMA, Colney Hatch Female Patient Casebooks, H12/CH/B/11/001 085; NRO, Male Patient Casebooks, NCLA/6/2/2/1-12; NRO Female Patient Casebooks, NCLA/6/2/1/1-13; GMCRO, Male Patient Casebooks, ADMM/2/1-16; GMRCO, ADMF/2/1-21; LRO, Male Patient Casebooks, QAM/6/6/1-34; LRO, Female Patient Casebooks, QAM/6/6/1-34; BLAS, Male Patient Casebooks, LF31/1-12; BLAS, Female Patient Casebooks, LF29/1-12

five asylums boys were admitted more regularly than girls. Explanations for the gender disparity are numerous. Anne Borsay has suggested that elderly males found themselves confined in workhouses because they were less domestically competent and 'less useful within the family division of labour where child care was a marketable commodity'.[28] It is possible that a similar argument can be applied to younger males also. For instance, David Wright suggested that harmless female cases could have been made useful in the home by providing childcare for younger siblings and undertaking household chores. He also speculates that with increased migration during the period, an absence of older siblings in the household may have created a crisis of care and made families more willing to seek institutional confinement for their children.[29] Developing this strand of investigation, a mentally impaired male child would have placed a long-term burden on the household economy. They were unlikely to be apprenticed or find regular work and would therefore be a substantial drain on family finances and often dependent on support from the poor law ratepayer into later life. The problem would be amplified when the child acted violently or was uncontrollable, a not uncommon occurrence.

Aside from gender differences, the children admitted to asylums formed a unique and distinct faction of the patient population because their congenital disabilities were not found frequently in adults. The American physician, Samuel G. Howe, described the most severe of these cases as masses of flesh and bone in human shape and went on to state that they 'are much below insects and so little above a sensitive plant'.[30] Perhaps less controversially for modern sensibilities, the prominent French physiologist and psychologist Edward Seguin, a proponent of education for those with mental disabilities and founder of a school for them in Paris in 1837, described idiots as those 'who know nothing, can do nothing, cannot even desire to do anything'.[31] Since then the concept of idiocy and its variants have evolved through numerous gradations and labels: feeble-minded, mentally deficient, retarded, and now in modern terminology learning disabled. Alienists thought cases of idiocy and imbecility were unsuitable admissions to the asylum, despite the legislative terminology of 1845, because they were incurable and generally harmless.[32] Due to their conditions it was thought that they were a low priority and occupied an inferior place.[33] For the Poor Law Medical Officer, the frontline in dealing with all pauper illness, idiots and imbeciles were often costly in terms of finance and time; on occasion these patients could be admitted to the asylum in order to ease this burden.[34] The techniques used to define idiot and imbecile patients in the process of certification is therefore particularly important. Whether their behaviour was constructed in a certain way designed to justify asylum admission particularly needs to be evaluated.

Bearing in mind legislative changes concerning asylums, particularly developments relating to idiocy, it is important to identify when children were admitted to the asylums and the symptoms that they were suffering from. Figure 2.1 demonstrates that more children were confined in asylums towards the end of the period, and that cases of idiocy and imbecility were admitted, peaking around 1890, regardless of their unsuitability. The reasons for increased admissions at this point in time are linked to increased institutional capacities, the rise in eugenic influence, and changes in regional welfare dynamics. The numbers did not explode, mainly because although asylum space was increasing it was still finite and in the

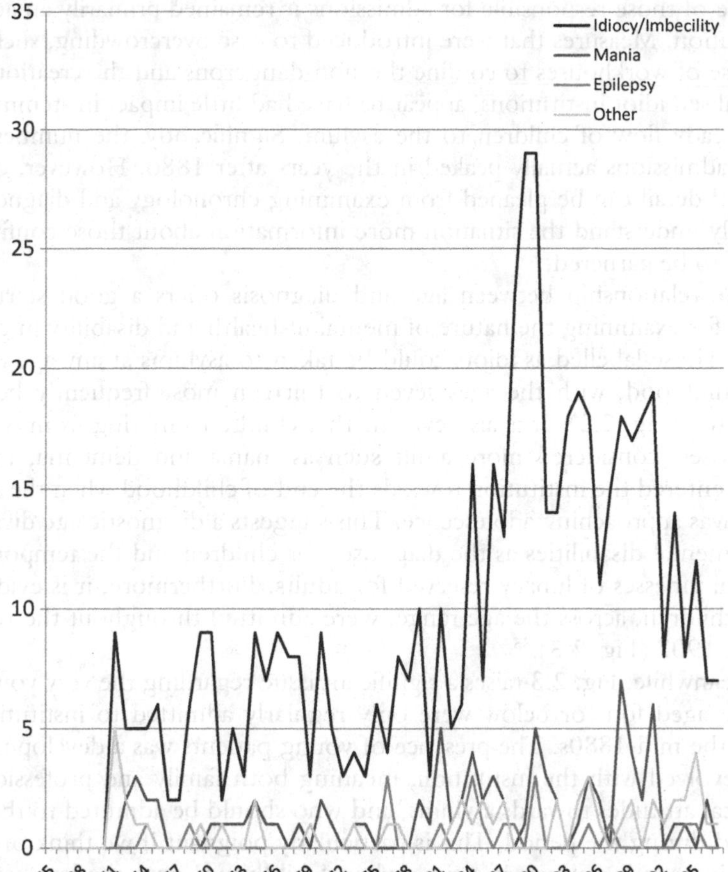

Fig. 2.1 Timeline of child admissions by diagnosis. *Source*: BCL, Male Patient Casebooks, MS344/12/2 & 2a, MS344/12/5, MS344/12/7-9, MS344/12/11-14, MS344/12/20-22, MS344/12/27; BCL, Female Patient Casebooks, MS344/12/41-47, MS344/12/49-51, MS344/12/53 & 54, MS344/12/56 & 57, MS344/12/60-63; BCL, Patient Index, MS344/11/1 & 2; LMA, Colney Hatch Male Patient Casebooks, H12/CH/B/13/001-61; LMA, Colney Hatch Female Patient Casebooks, H12/CH/B/11/001-085; NRO, Male Patient Casebooks, NCLA/6/2/2/1-12; NRO Female Patient Casebooks, NCLA/6/2/1/1-13; GMCRO, Male Patient Casebooks, ADMM/2/1-16; GMRCO, ADMF/2/1-21; LRO, Male Patient Casebooks, QAM/6/6/1-34; LRO, Female Patient Casebooks, QAM/6/6/1-34; BLAS, Male Patient Casebooks, LF31/1-12; BLAS, Female Patient Casebooks, LF29/1-12

psyche of those responsible for admissions it remained primarily an adult institution. Measures that were introduced to ease overcrowding, such as the use of workhouses to confine the non-dangerous and the creation of specialised idiot institutions, appear to have had little impact in stemming the steady flow of children to the asylum. Significantly, the number of idiot admissions actually peaked in the years after 1886. However, only limited detail can be gleaned from examining chronology and diagnosis, to fully understand the situation more information about those confined needs to be garnered.

The relationship between age and diagnosis offers a good starting point for examining the nature of mental ill-health and disability in children. Those labelled as idiots could be taken to asylums at any age during childhood, with the ages seven to thirteen most frequently being admitted (Fig. 2.2). It is also evident that children suffering from other diagnoses, considered more adult such as mania and dementia, most likely entered the institution towards the end of childhood when the sufferer was approaching adolescence. This suggests a diagnostic age divide, with mental disabilities as the diagnoses for children and the temporary mental illnesses of lunacy reserved for adults. Furthermore, it is evident that children, across the age range, were admitted throughout the years 1845–1907 (Fig. 2.3).[35]

Meanwhile, Fig. 2.3 raises a significant issue regarding the very young. Those aged four or below were only regularly admitted to institutions from the mid-1880s. The presence of young patients was a development that evolved with the institution, meaning both family and professional medical attitudes towards asylums, and who should be admitted to them, shifted during the period. This is particularly poignant if we think of the late-nineteenth century as a time when 'childhood', in a modern sense, emerged and infants were beginning to be socially and legally protected.[36] An enthralling paradox existed where the children of the poor were being accepted as a vulnerable social group in need of security, but at the same time those with a mental impairment were occupying an increasing proportion of asylum capacity, alongside potentially dangerous adults. This situation, however, might be unsurprising if we consider the nascent concept of childhood as only applying to the fit, healthy, and potentially productive, and leaving those that fall outside of this model to get by in whatever means necessary. Developments such as elementary education amplified the impairments of those not fitting the established model of

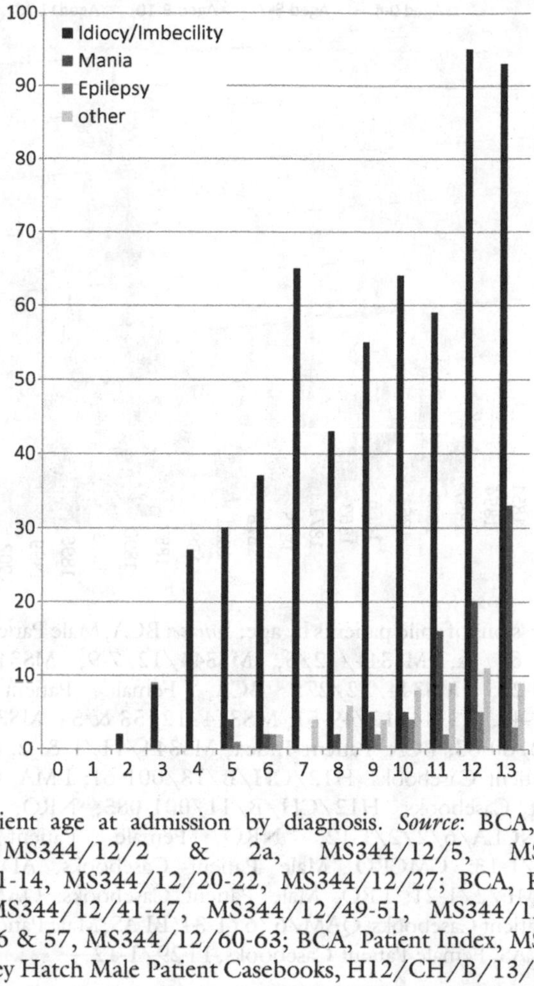

Fig. 2.2 Patient age at admission by diagnosis. *Source*: BCA, Male Patient Casebooks, MS344/12/2 & 2a, MS344/12/5, MS344/12/7-9, MS344/12/11-14, MS344/12/20-22, MS344/12/27; BCA, Female Patient Casebooks, MS344/12/41-47, MS344/12/49-51, MS344/12/53 & 54, MS344/12/56 & 57, MS344/12/60-63; BCA, Patient Index, MS344/11/1 & 2; LMA, Colney Hatch Male Patient Casebooks, H12/CH/B/13/001-61; LMA, Colney Hatch Female Patient Casebooks, H12/CH/B/11/001-085; NRO, Male Patient Casebooks, NCLA/6/2/2/1-12; NRO Female Patient Casebooks, NCLA/6/2/1/1-13; GMCRO, Male Patient Casebooks, ADMM/2/1-16; GMCRO, ADMF/2/1-21; LRO, Male Patient Casebooks, QAM/6/6/1-34; LRO, Female Patient Casebooks, QAM/6/6/1-34; BLAS, Male Patient Casebooks, LF31/1-12; BLAS, Female Patient Casebooks, LF29/1-12

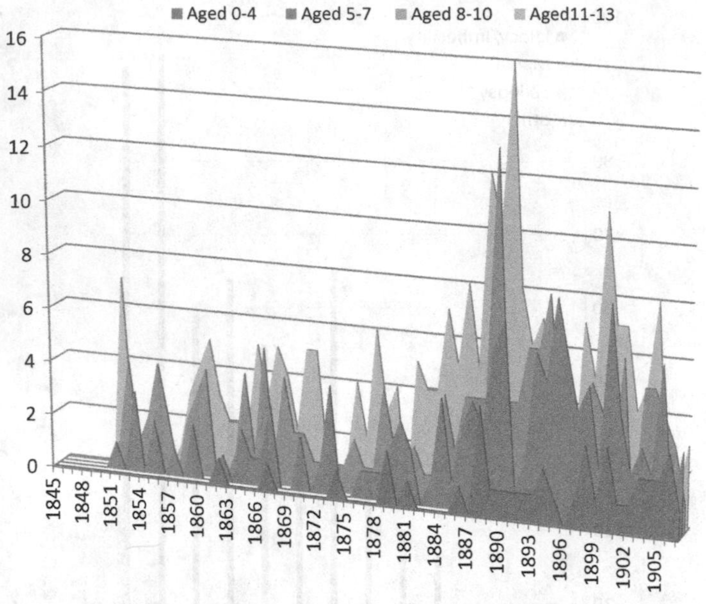

Fig. 2.3 Admissions of child patients by age. *Source*: BCA, Male Patient Casebooks, MS344/12/2 & 2a, MS344/12/5, MS344/12/7-9, MS344/12/11-14, MS344/12/20-22, MS344/12/27; BCA, Female Patient Casebooks, MS344/12/41-47, MS344/12/49-51, MS344/12/53 & 54, MS344/12/56 & 57, MS344/12/60-63; BCA, Patient Index, MS344/11/1 & 2; LMA, Colney Hatch Male Patient Casebooks, H12/CH/B/13/001-61; LMA, Colney Hatch Female Patient Casebooks, H12/CH/B/11/001-085; NRO, Male Patient Casebooks, NCLA/6/2/2/1-12; NRO Female Patient Casebooks, NCLA/6/2/1/1-13; GMCRO, Male Patient Casebooks, ADMM/2/1-16; GMRCO, ADMF/2/1-21; LRO, Male Patient Casebooks, QAM/6/6/1-34; LRO, Female Patient Casebooks, QAM/6/6/1-34; BLAS, Male Patient Casebooks, LF31/1-12; BLAS, Female Patient Casebooks, LF29/1-12

perfection and, for the first time, they became subject to wider scrutiny and assessment than ever before.

Indeed, by the end of the nineteenth century educational failure was the most important yardstick used to define mental incapacity. Parents and teachers used those visible to them as measures by which to judge a child's development.[37] A number of children admitted to asylums were described as being unable to learn or play with other children, were threatening to others in school, or were judged to be not as 'sharp' as their peers. For instance, when Amos Tullet, aged twelve, entered the Berrywood Asylum in 1890 it was noted that 'he will not play with the other boys';[38] Alfred Hamp entered the same institution nine years later, being 'always regarded as queer, went to school until 3 months ago ... he has been the butt of the other boys for 4 or 5 years';[39] and when Alice Popper was admitted to the Three Counties asylum, aged only four, in 1874, it was recorded that '[she] cannot learn her letters or anything else'.[40] These children demonstrate that education developed as an intellectual and social apparatus to identify, and eventually further, difference in mental capability in the years following 1870. Also, significantly, this was the point in time when family roles of identification and diagnosis began to diminish in favour of professional, state constructed, ideas and causes of mental impairment.[41]

Explaining the Causes of Child Insanity

Asylum patient case histories were created by asylum physicians and recorded in casebooks, these narratives were the place where causative explanations for mental illnesses and disabilities were documented. By exploring causes and classifications for child insanity during the second half of the nineteenth century the importance of family testimonies will become apparent and the nature of historical child mental impairment becomes clearer.

The aetiological circumstances surrounding insanity in children can be grouped into three categories. These are hereditary, acquired, and developmental and represent a departure from the experience of adult patients whose causes were divided between the moral, physical, and, as the period progressed, 'impaired'.[42] Ideas of 'impairment' were linked to hereditary explanations and incurability, while those with moral and physical causes, in the right circumstances, could recover. So the split between chronicity and temporary conditions persisted. The asylum was thus a paradoxical institution; on the one hand it was curative for those with non-hereditary causes, on the other it was custodial and designed to stem social decline and improve productivity.[43] Children fit with both purposes, but their conditions, unlike adult patients, could not be ascribed to life-cycle events such as old age, strokes, or lifestyle choices such as intemperance or sexual promiscuity. The young had no such baggage and the causes of their insanity had to be sought elsewhere. A total of 313 children (41 %) were assigned a cause for their condition.[44] This is a significant amount, but a large number received no explanation as to the onset of their impairment. These tended to have their causes listed as 'unknown', 'congenital', or 'due to epilepsy'. Of the 460 cases with no explanation there were 235 (52 %) diagnosed as idiots or epileptics from birth.

Contemporary physicians most often believed that the causes of idiocy and imbecility were hereditary or a result of parental actions prior to birth. Samuel Howe argued that idiocy occurred in children because parents 'violated the natural laws of man'.[45] These violations ranged from illegitimacy, drunkenness, vagrancy and criminality, to attempted abortion or intermarriage, all of which were perceived crimes of the lower orders. Similarly, Edward Seguin argued that the causes of idiocy were hereditary, but went further by suggesting that blame was maternal by contending that the mother was usually 'under-fed [and] in poverty herself'.[46] Such a view exemplifies the contemporary belief in the intrinsic links between poverty and insanity.[47] There were 166 (22 %) children with hereditary links to insanity and they accounted for 53 % of all causes given. These family ties were varied and occasionally obscure, ranging from the insanity of immediate family members, such as parents or grandparents, to more tenuous links of maternal or paternal great uncles and aunts. For medical men it was of paramount importance to establish the medical history of the family when admitting children. Therefore on casefiles we see statements such as: 'father an imbecile', 'hereditary maternal aunt [insane]', and 'hereditary paternal grandfather and aunt [in asylum]'.[48]

Of those assigned a hereditary cause, 102 (61 %) were described as congenital or suffering from their condition since birth. These children were spread across the age range with the youngest being four years old and the eldest thirteen. When looking at those at the older end of the age scale there must have been a concerted effort to care for children in the domestic sphere prior to institutionalisation or, alternatively, they must have been refused treatment consistently before finally being admitted. The non-congenital hereditary insane suffered with their conditions for on average ten months before admission to the asylum, only a fraction of the time experienced by congenital cases.

The second most frequent causative explanation related to those who had acquired their conditions. Acquisition, it was thought, could occur in a variety of ways, from a shock to the mother during pregnancy, accidents that caused cerebral injury, illness, and even sunstroke. There were 127 (17%) children that fell within this category, accounting for a total of 41 % of all recorded causes. Breaking this down further, 44 (35%) came as a result of shock or fright; 59 (46%) through injury; and 24 (19%) were believed to have been acquired as a result of illnesses such as measles, whooping cough, influenza or typhoid.[49] Some emblematic cases are those of: Stephen Webster admitted aged thirteen to the Berrywood Asylum in 1882, he had suffered an injury to the head that was caused by a plough three years previously;[50] William Brazier admitted to Berrywood in 1900 at the age of twelve, he had been found unconscious following a fall from a tree, subsequently he started suffering from 'fits';[51] at Three Counties Asylum, Bertram Warring suffered a 'traumatic' head injury prior to admission in 1883, he was aged seven;[52] Ernest Morgan, aged twelve, was admitted in 1874 to Three Counties, his mother had received a fright whilst pregnant; and Agnes Reeve, at Three Counties, it was noted, had the cause of sunstroke recorded for her mania.[53] Furthermore, in the Birmingham asylum Samuel Gardiner was admitted at the age of eleven in 1907, his insanity was 'caused by measles' and Florry Wright, aged ten, had the cause of her insanity recorded in 1889 as a fright to the mother during pregnancy.[54]

In comparison to hereditary causes only thirty-three (26%) of acquired cases were described as congenital. If those that had suffered frights or shock in pregnancy are removed from the equation then the total reduces to seven (6%), demonstrating further the role of parents, particularly the mother and her constitution, in shaping explanations for childhood mental disability. Those with non-congenital acquired conditions on average waited just under four years before their families sought asylum admission. The duration, however, is distorted somewhat by the wide variations in the length of time children displayed symptoms in this category; the shortest amount of time before admission being just three days after the child suffered a fall,[55] and the longest eleven years.[56]

The final explanation was found in the developmental stages of childhood. Although they number considerably fewer than the previous two categories they are still an important element for understanding contemporaneous attitudes. Examples of developmental causes totalled just nineteen or 3 % of the overall sample, but they featured in all of the institutions examined. Children in this category were either at the younger end of the age group, for example those that were caused by teething accounted for fourteen cases (eight males and six females)—these had usually suffered febrile seizures—or at the older end of the scale where five cases, all of them girls, that had the onset of puberty recorded as a cause. This suggests a fear of reproduction, or the potential reproduction of individuals that were mentally weak, a cornerstone of eugenic anxieties about the feeble-minded towards the end of the nineteenth century. On average the length of time before admission for the developmental strand was, in line with hereditary and acquired causes, 4.1 years. What is clear is that the child with hereditary links to insanity, but had not displayed symptoms from birth, found its way to the asylum much quicker than acquired or developmental cases; emphasising the importance of family and the child's background in the process of identifying mental disability in the young.

For non-hereditary cases admission to the asylum was neither a fast nor first choice option. Unfortunately, asylum records are not definitive personal accounts and do not provide complete access to family circumstances and hence often fail to explain why admission occurred when it did. The significant average length of time before admission can be interpreted in a number of ways. Firstly, families were willing to care for their insane children and they sought help only after a substantial amount of time or they suffered a change in domestic circumstances.[57] This could be considered the positive approach to confinement. Conversely, it could be that the treatment of these children had been avoided or neglected by families, or medical men, or both.[58] Both of these views are equally valid and examples have already featured. The nature and scope of asylum documents and the lack of family records for paupers make it difficult to develop these strands of analysis further. The experience of children with supposed 'medical' causes for their condition demonstrate that they were not despatched to the asylum at the first opportunity by their families.

Causes were most frequently recorded from the 1880s (Fig. 2.4). It had been assumed that from the mid-nineteenth century, as chronicity and incurability became more common, the causes, classifications, and treatments of these conditions became unnecessary.[59] Not only was this a time when the diagnosis of mental disabilities was increasing, it was also apparent that the proportion of the general population suffering from insanity was rising—the overcrowding in most county asylums is testament to this and in 1894 the London County Council lamented an inability to stem the average rise of 400 lunatics per year in the metropolis.[60] Explanations for this increase, both for children and adults, were sought in an intellectual climate influenced by Darwin's *On the Origin of Species* published in 1859. The influential and controversial principle of the survival of the fittest was applied to human populations by Darwin's cousin Sir Francis Galton. He posited that human abilities were inherited and in 1883 he

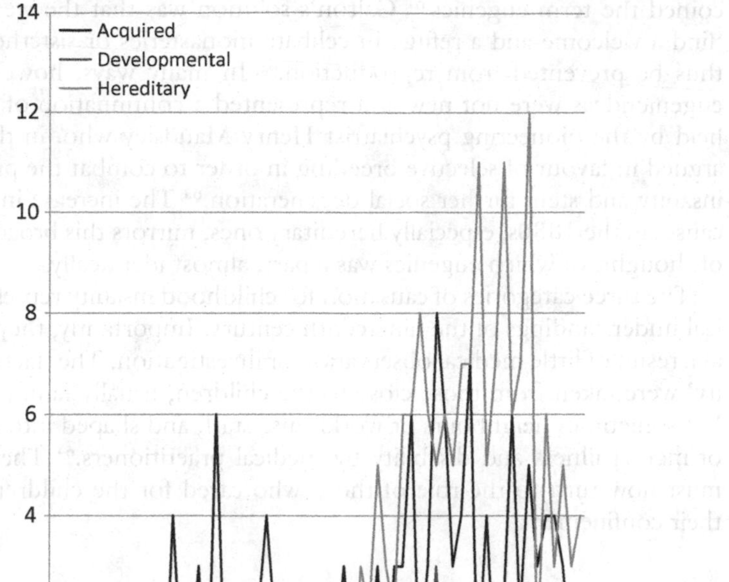

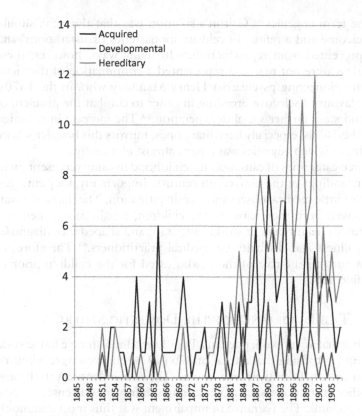

Fig. 2.4 Child admission dates by causative explanation. *Source*: BCA, Male Patient Casebooks, MS344/12/2 & 2a, MS344/12/5, MS344/12/7-9, MS344/12/11-14, MS344/12/20-22, MS344/12/27; BCA, Female Patient Casebooks, MS344/12/41-47, MS344/12/49-51, MS344/12/53 & 54, MS344/12/56 & 57, MS344/12/60-63; BCA, Patient Index, MS344/11/1 & 2; LMA, Colney Hatch Male Patient Casebooks, H12/CH/B/13/001-61; LMA, Colney Hatch Female Patient Casebooks, H12/CH/B/11/001-085; NRO, Male Patient Casebooks, NCLA/6/2/2/1-12; NRO Female Patient Casebooks, NCLA/6/2/1/1-13; GMCRO, Male Patient Casebooks, ADMM/2/1-16; GMCRO, ADMF/2/1-21; LRO, Male Patient Casebooks, QAM/6/6/1-34; LRO, Female Patient Casebooks, QAM/6/6/1-34; BLAS, Male Patient Casebooks, LF31/1-12; BLAS, Female Patient Casebooks, LF29/1-12

coined the term eugenics.[61] Galton's solution was that the weak should 'find a welcome and a refuge in celibate monasteries or sisterhoods' and thus be prevented from reproduction.[62] In many ways, however, these eugenic ideas were not new and represented a continuation of the views held by the pioneering psychiatrist Henry Maudsley who, in the 1870s, argued in favour of selective breeding in order to combat the problem of insanity and stem further social degeneration.[63] The increase in recorded causes in the 1880s, especially hereditary ones, mirrors this broader school of thought, of which eugenics was a part, almost identically.

The three categories of causation for childhood insanity represent medical understandings of the nineteenth century. Importantly, they emerged as a result of little medical observation or investigation. The 'facts of insanity' were taken from those close to the children, usually family members but sometimes neighbours or workhouse staff, and shaped into diagnoses of mental illness and disability by medical practitioners.[64] Therefore we must now turn to the role of those who cared for the children prior to their confinement.

The Importance of the Domestic Sphere

Considering that asylums operated in a Poor Law administrative framework, it is, perhaps, surprising that a total of 376 (49 %) children were admitted to asylums directly from their own homes. The remainder went to the asylum via other institutions, such as workhouses, infirmaries, licensed houses, and other asylums. The narrative of impairment was thus most commonly developed within the domestic sphere and presented to the medical establishment where it was 'medicalised' by those with perceived expert knowledge. Evidently, childhood mental disability, as a construction, was a result of a cultural negotiation between lay and expert opinion.[65] Certificates of Insanity even contained a substantial space where 'others' were able to record notable facts about the case. This gave family members the opportunity to make their case for asylum admission, and when filtered through the medical opinion of the professional recording the information it was often shaped to support a particular diagnosis.[66] Consequently, we are exposed to those examples where familial contributions were most convincing and influential, and access to situations where family comments were considered unhelpful, unimportant, or inaccurate are more limited.

There are, however, numerous illustrations of the domestic sphere permeating the process of diagnosis. George Canfield was admitted to Three

Counties in 1876. He was said to be 'very restless, spiteful to his brother and sisters not safe to be left alone for one minute'.[67] Similarly, Sydney Virtue a patient in Colney Hatch from 1898, received a diagnosis heavily influenced by his mother who stated 'he is very violent at times, uses dreadful language, molests and spits in peoples [sic] faces in the streets'. The professional statements accompanying this testimony echoed these comments but in a medical vernacular. Virtue was said to be 'deficient in manner, restless, excitable and dangerous to himself ... requires constant watching'.[68] Such examples demonstrate the centrality of family testimony in constructing child insanity. This is reinforced further when considering the causes presented above. Whether the explanation for insanity was perceived to be hereditary, acquired or developmental, the facts used to make this judgement originated in the domestic sphere. In essence, lay opinion presented the case for child insanity and the medical establishment validated it.[69] Bearing this situation in mind, an examination of how and when the asylum was accessed is essential to better understand the experience of these children and their families.

A revisionist school of historians has argued that families used the asylum to deposit their unwanted, unproductive or awkward members.[70] When looking at the children in the five asylums used here there were 418 (54 %) that had suffered with their conditions all of their lives and had no record of interaction with the medical profession before being taken to the asylum. Such a high figure might suggest that asylums were resorted to at the first instance by families, but it has already been demonstrated that the average length of time before admission could be substantial, and thus a better explanation is required. The counter-revisionist school argued that when families sought out the provision of the asylum they did so 'strategically'.[71] These scholars have suggested that the greatest strain on household economies came after child-bearing had ceased, but before children contributed more to the household than they took from it.[72] Due to the nature of pauper records identifying any strategic use of the asylum by families is complex and the extant medical records of the asylum offer little insight into the domestic dynamic. The length of time that child patients spent in asylums could be considered a crucial element in determining how the asylum was utilised by families. The core issue being whether children were the unwanted and long-term patients or whether there is evidence of short-term, strategic, asylum solutions utilised by families.[73]

The average period of confinement for children in the asylums was four years and five months. This, however, masks a multitude of experiences and one standard deviation from the norm was seven years, so it is evident that plenty of children were confined for much longer than the average. Exploring further, those that fit within the causative framework remained in the institution on average for just under two years and eleven months. In this instance, one standard deviation from the norm was just over six years and demonstrates that whilst those with causative explanations were confined for less time than the whole sample, the length of stay was still considerable. While average durations were lengthy, not all children were long-stay patients in the asylum. However, that does not mean that they eventually returned to their homes and previous lives when they departed the institution.

In order to demonstrate any strategic use of the asylum the destinations that children departed to require examination. If the asylum was accessed as part of a family's welfare strategy it would be expected that discharge at request of 'friends', a term used to describe family members or those close to them, or recovery would be the most frequently recorded reason for leaving, in order to facilitate a return to the domestic environment. However, this was fairly uncommon and removal to 'friends' only accounted for thirty-one cases. Moreover, children admitted to asylums most commonly died inside them, not the desired outcome if the institution was accessed as a temporary measure. Therefore if asylums were used strategically at the point of admission then families were incapable, or less active, in seeking the discharge of their children following confinement. Even when children were not long-stay patients they were unlikely to return home after being admitted to the asylum. Nevertheless, using patient casefile analysis it is still possible to identify some strategic use of the asylum.

The catalyst in roughly 10 % of child admissions to asylums was not their mental conditions, but the somatic illness of a parent or carer. These illnesses were usually those that affected the poorer elements of society, such as the degenerative lung conditions phthisis and consumption.[74] A parent suffering from latter stage phthisis would have struggled to provide and care for their children. In addition, medical opinion in the mid-nineteenth century linked insanity and lung diseases and unintentionally promoted children as prime candidates for admission.[75] Consequently, family ties, or the lack of them, to tuberculosis, phthisis, and consumption regularly featured in the certification of children. When John Scott was admitted to the asylum in Northampton, from his grandfather's home, it was because his parents were both consumptive.[76] In Birmingham, Tom Skirrow was admitted to the asylum following the death of his grandparents with whom he lived. His mother was stated to also be dead and his father absconded. He eventually died from phthisis in the institution.[77] Looking more widely at childhood experience, lung diseases were the most prolific killers of children in the asylums, accounting for 103 of the 353 (29 %) deaths that occurred.[78] The asylum thus became a destination for children suffering with a mental impairment when families faced domestic shifts that affected their ability to provide care.[79] In these situations familial attitudes towards insane children can be considered a positive and the asylum was used as a last resort to provide safety and security, rather than the punitive institution of the workhouse (Fig. 2.5).

Patient casebooks provide some insight into the attitudes and thoughts of families towards their mentally impaired children. Modern medical records are designed to be objective and state medical facts, they are not designed to record emotions. Their nineteenth-century counterparts were, however, much more fluid in what they documented and while often they gave an impression of distant and uncaring families they also provide glimpses of parental feelings towards children. For example, in the Berrywood Asylum casebooks a newspaper obituary is attached to Walter Quinnell's casefile. The insertion reports the death of 'Walter, beloved son of Daniel and Edith Quinnell, after a long and painful illness, aged 7'.[80] While the wording might appear typical of this kind of public notification, the fact that the family went to the cost and effort of making it is a clear sign of compassion for and sadness at the death of a family member that had suffered from a mental disability and been treated in an asylum. The presence of the obituary on the correct page for the patient, who had been discharged from the asylum two years previously, also shows a certain degree of compassion on the part of the institution. We are, however, unaware who was responsible for the placement of the cutting. The family may have sent it to the asylum to inform them of the passing of their son or it may have been found in the newspaper by a member of staff that had treated the child.

Similarly, and again in Northamptonshire, Sidney Carrington's family described their feelings on the death of their son in a heartfelt letter to asylum. The family stated that they 'would like to thank you for your kindness to our dear Sidney and for your kind sympathy in our great loss for we did love him so much'.[81] Again these are hardly sentiments of families that saw insane members as unwanted or a burden. At Colney Hatch, Henrietta Lamb's parents wrote to the asylum asking when they could

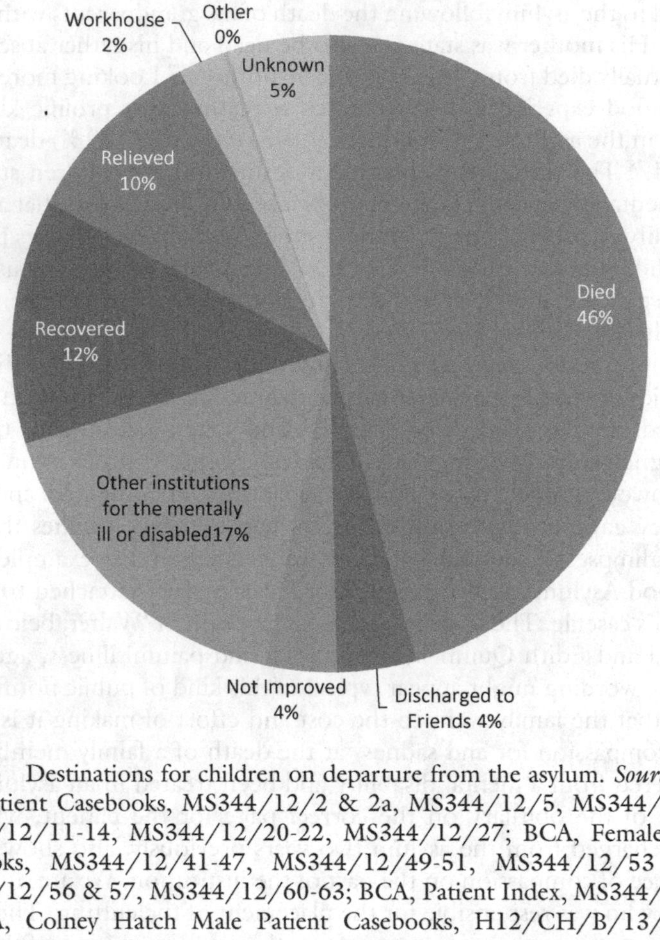

Fig. 2.5 Destinations for children on departure from the asylum. *Source*: BCA, Male Patient Casebooks, MS344/12/2 & 2a, MS344/12/5, MS344/12/7-9, MS344/12/11-14, MS344/12/20-22, MS344/12/27; BCA, Female Patient Casebooks, MS344/12/41-47, MS344/12/49-51, MS344/12/53 & 54, MS344/12/56 & 57, MS344/12/60-63; BCA, Patient Index, MS344/11/1 & 2; LMA, Colney Hatch Male Patient Casebooks, H12/CH/B/13/001-61; LMA, Colney Hatch Female Patient Casebooks, H12/CH/B/11/001-085; NRO, Male Patient Casebooks, NCLA/6/2/2/1-12; NRO Female Patient Casebooks, NCLA/6/2/1/1-13; GMCRO, Male Patient Casebooks, ADMM/2/1-16; GMCRO, ADMF/2/1-21; LRO, Male Patient Casebooks, QAM/6/6/1-34; LRO, Female Patient Casebooks, QAM/6/6/1-34; BLAS, Male Patient Casebooks, LF31/1-12; BLAS, Female Patient Casebooks, LF29/1-12

visit, displaying a clear desire to see their child even though they lived at a distance.[82] The difficulty with attempting to identify family emotions towards insane children is that these issues rarely permeated the medical documents. It is thus easy to deduce a lack of care or compassion and assume that children were deposited in the asylum because they were a burden and unloved.

The Prism of Idiocy

Idiocy was the most common diagnosis for children admitted to the asylum during this period. Three-quarters of the children in the five asylums (76 % of males and 74 % of females) were diagnosed as idiots or imbeciles.[83] These two conditions are examined together because they were often synonymous within the medical lexicon of the nineteenth century. In 1875 George Grabham, the Medical Superintendent at Earlswood Idiot Asylum, acknowledged the similarities of the two conditions by suggesting imbecility should be considered a milder form of idiocy that developed during infancy rather than being congenital.[84] These similarities were reinforced further when George Shuttleworth illustrated the distinctions between lunatics and idiots and imbeciles. He treated idiots and imbeciles as a single group, separate from the temporary condition of lunacy and supported Grabham's view of imbecility being a milder form of idiocy.[85] The language of insanity is important when dealing with idiocy because it was an all-encompassing and catch-all term. There is not a single example of these mental impairments but a whole spectrum of symptoms that amalgamated to construct them. A point reinforced by the conceptual shift, a consequence of eugenic influence, in how idiocy and mental impairment was observed during the nineteenth century. During the period it has been argued that idiots were no longer viewed as qualitatively different from the norm, but instead came to be seen as distinct and separate from the 'normal' population.[86] Here the validity of such a claim will be tested.[87]

To do justice to the spectrum of behaviours, actions, and symptoms that combined to form the conditions of idiocy and imbecility they will be further subdivided in order to provide more nuanced examples. These subcategories—the harmless, the epileptic, and the dangerous—reflect the most frequently recorded descriptions. A number of emblematic case studies will demonstrate standard models for each subdivision. Anomalies or exceptional variants for each will be presented once the 'norm' has been established.

The most common subgroups admitted to asylums were the harmless and epileptic (Table 2.2). Cases such as these, it has been assumed, were not sent to asylums. Anne Borsay stated that harmless lunatics remained outside the institution with 'only those considered difficult and dangerous being dispatched to the asylum'.[88] A view echoed by Wright who argued that the mentally disabled were only sent to asylums if they became violent or unruly.[89] We see in Table 2.2, however, that harmless and epileptic cases of idiocy were confined in larger numbers than the dangerous and violent. Traditionally, it has been argued that at the beginning of the period some of these cases may have been admitted because asylum medical superintendents did not want to cede medical responsibility to lay authorities, even though they were unenthusiastic about incurable idiots clogging up space in institutions.[90] Yet, moving to Fig. 2.6, it is evident that the majority of harmless and epileptic cases were admitted to asylums much later in the period, with the two decades from 1880 witnessing most admissions probably in response to the nascent eugenic belief in segregating the mentally deficient.

Of these harmless patients, John Harvey, aged ten, was admitted to the Colney Hatch Asylum in 1852. His casefile states he was in good physical health, the duration of his 'disease' was five years and there was no

Table 2.2 Admission numbers for subcategories of mental disability

	Birmingham M-F	*Colney Hatch M-F*	*Manchester M-F*	*Northampton M-F*	*Three Counties M-F*	*Total M-F*
Harmless	8–8	30–17	6–5	56–38	32–15	132–83
Epileptic	9–5	45–17	11–4	33–21	26–12	121–59
Dangerous	4–3	27–3	3–9	21–9	11–9	66–33
Ep & Dangerous	8–4	12–1	4–2	17–16	6–15	47–38
Total	29–20	114–38	24–20	127–84	75–51	369–213

Source: BCA, Male Patient Casebooks, MS344/12/2 & 2a, MS344/12/5, MS344/12/7-9, MS344/12/11-14, MS344/12/20-22, MS344/12/27; BCA, Female Patient Casebooks, MS344/12/41-47, MS344/12/49-51, MS344/12/53 & 54, MS344/12/56 & 57, MS344/12/60-63; BCA, Patient Index, MS344/11/1 & 2; LMA, Colney Hatch Male Patient Casebooks, H12/CH/B/13/001-61; LMA, Colney Hatch Female Patient Casebooks, H12/CH/B/11/001-085; NRO, Male Patient Casebooks, NCLA/6/2/2/1-12; NRO Female Patient Casebooks, NCLA/6/2/1/1-13; GMCRO, Male Patient Casebooks, ADMM/2/1-16; GMCRO, ADMF/2/1-21; LRO, Male Patient Casebooks, QAM/6/6/1-34; LRO, Female Patient Casebooks, QAM/6/6/1-34; BLAS, Male Patient Casebooks, LF31/1-12; BLAS, Female Patient Casebooks, LF29/1-12

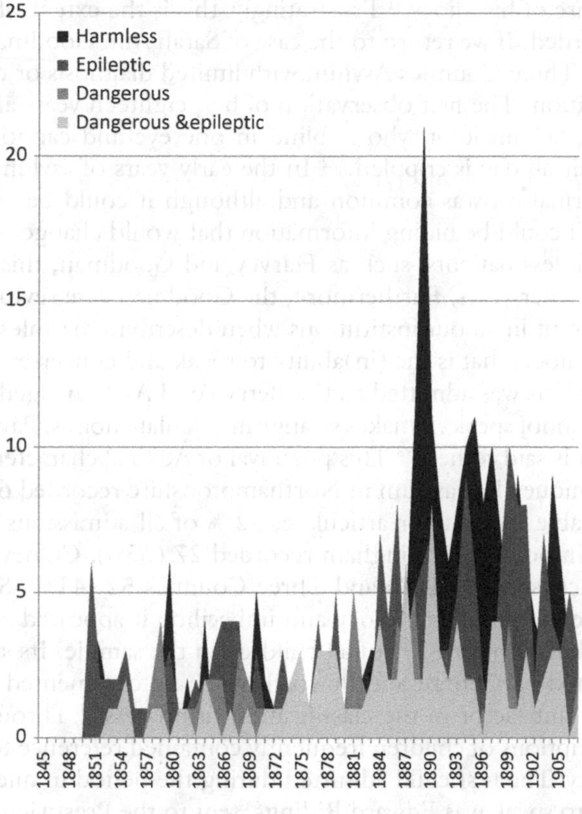

Fig. 2.6 Years of admission for idiot and imbecile child patients. Source: BCA, Male Patient Casebooks, MS344/12/2 & 2a, MS344/12/5, MS344/12/7-9, MS344/12/11-14, MS344/12/20-22, MS344/12/27; BCA, Female Patient Casebooks, MS344/12/41-47, MS344/12/49-51, MS344/12/53 & 54, MS344/12/56 & 57, MS344/12/60-63; BCA, Patient Index, MS344/11/1 & 2; LMA, Colney Hatch Male Patient Casebooks, H12/CH/B/13/001-61; LMA, Colney Hatch Female Patient Casebooks, H12/CH/B/11/001-085; NRO, Male Patient Casebooks, NCLA/6/2/2/1-12; NRO Female Patient Casebooks, NCLA/6/2/1/1-13; GMCRO, Male Patient Casebooks, ADMM/2/1-16; GMRCO, ADMF/2/1-21; LRO, Male Patient Casebooks, QAM/6/6/1-34; LRO, Female Patient Casebooks, QAM/6/6/1-34; BLAS, Male Patient Casebooks, LF31/1-12; BLAS, Female Patient Casebooks, LF29/1-12

assigned cause of his idiocy.[91] Frustratingly, this is the extent of the information recorded. If we return to the case of Sarah Ann Goodman, she was admitted to Three Counties Asylum with limited diagnosis or description of her condition. The first observation of her, eighteen years after admission, stated, 'a thin idiot who is blind in one eye and cannot talk. Sits still in a chair all day is crippled.'[92] In the early years of asylumdom such limited information was common and although it could be argued that limited detail could be hiding information that would change our perceptions of harmless patients, such as Harvey and Goodman, this is not the situation for later years. Furthermore, the Goodman case reveals a theme that is recurrent in all our institutions when describing harmless congenital cases of idiocy; that is the (in)ability to speak and converse.

Mabel Adkins was admitted to the Berrywood Asylum, aged six, it was stated 'she cannot speak … makes strange inarticulate noises. Pays no attention to what is said to her.'[93] This portrayal of Adkins' characteristics is by no means unique. The asylum in Northamptonshire recorded 68 children as being unable to speak or articulate, 32 % of all admissions diagnosed as idiots or imbeciles; Birmingham recorded 27 (55%), Colney Hatch 61 (39%), Manchester 19 (43%) and Three Counties 52 (41%). Speech was a key feature in identifying idiocy and imbecility; it appeared as a characteristic at admission for 32 % of all children in the sample. Its significance was also noted by George Shuttleworth when he commented on speech as an important factor in the classification of process.[94] Throughout the period descriptions of children frequently contained reference to their linguistic ability. The first child admitted during the period in question with an inability to speak was Edward Ridings, sent to the Prestwich Asylum in Manchester on 13 February 1851.[95] The last was Jane Denifer, aged four, admitted to Three Counties Asylum on 19 October 1907.[96] Significantly, the inability to speak or articulate remained a stable method of description for all institutions across the years 1851–1907.

Evidently, not all children with a diagnosis of idiocy were admitted with an inability to converse, for those who could speak their linguistic dexterity was still used to determine their condition. When Eliza Spencer Perry, aged six, was admitted to Three Counties Asylum in 1905, it was stated she 'doesn't speak when spoken to but makes grunting noises'.[97] At Northampton, Arthur Harry White was admitted in 1889. He was able to answer simple questions and could tell his name at admission but it was recorded on his case file that 'his conversation is incoherent'.[98] Incoherence and the inability to answer 'simple' questions featured regularly . The statement about White establishes a link between incoherence and a judgement of a child's 'intelligence', another pillar in constructing the idiot or imbecile child.

Intelligence was not assessed in an objective or uniform way but varied depending on the child and institution. Arthur White could answer 'simple questions', but we have no idea what those questions were, so judging their simplicity from our viewpoint is impossible. Constance Watson, at Three Counties Asylum, was able to answer the 'simple questions' put to her but she could not count, tell her age, or day of the week; again, the nature of the simple questions elude us, but we are afforded a greater insight into her mental abilities.[99] The case notes of John McCormack, aged twelve, reveal some of the potential lines of questioning children faced at admission; it was recorded that he did not know the difference between a six-pence and a penny.[100] Other children such as John Tanner and Sidney Bishop at Northampton,[101] Jacob Gaffey at Manchester,[102] Louisa Barley, Rhoda Key and Frederick Lawrence at Colney Hatch,[103] and Harriet Stocker at Three Counties were asked to read or write, list the days of the week, or name their family members but there was no standardised line of investigation.

A small minority of children that were confined as idiots bucked the trend and displayed some levels of intelligence or education when admitted. These were not representative of Howe's 'flesh and bone in human shape'. There was, however, a fine line between the patient that was beyond mental improvement and the patient that displayed some intelligence. For example, Ernest Cross admitted to the Northamptonshire asylum was said to be 'devoid of ordinary intelligence, inability to understand simple questions. Can count and tell the story of his father running away from his mother.'[104] Ideas of 'ordinary intelligence' and 'understanding simple questions' were of course subjective. Cross would have been asked about his family and retold the story of his father—could this not be seen as an answer to a simple question? Joseph Albert Harris, admitted to Northamptonshire aged eight, displayed 'ordinary intelligence' when admitted; he was said to be able to articulate many words in an intelligent way.[105] In the same institution, Sidney Bishop was said to be, somewhat oxymoronically, 'a smart, quick child to be dumb'. He could tell the days of the week and name all of his family members; however, he suffered from regular epileptic seizures which help to explain his admission.[106] Ellen Tarry, also admitted to Northamptonshire, was a 'child with a fair amount of intelligence, answers questions sensibly... Can write very well.'[107] Within the broad characteristics of idiocy there were devices used to identify, judge and label a child's condition. These varied between the different subcategories of idiocy, further highlighting the fluidity of the condition. For instance, Alice Popper admitted to Three Counties Asylum was described as 'an idiot, but not apparently of a bad type'.[108] This, however, did not mean that she displayed signs of intelligence like Joseph Harris, Sidney Bishop, or Ellen Tarry.

In 1837, the influential alienist W.A.F. Browne stated that 'there are gradations in the scale of idiocy. Certain individuals advance farther towards maturity of the mind than others, and yet fall short of what our intellectual nature is intended to be.'[109] Child asylum patients offer evidence as to these perceived gradations in the condition of idiocy. Popper's Medical Certificate recorded 'in reply to all questions her answer is no, no, no. She cannot learn her letters or anything else.' Except for the statement stating she is not a 'bad' type of idiot there is very little to judge how she differed from other cases of idiocy. Similarly, Annie Clarke, George Buckby and Kate Robinson, all admitted to Northamptonshire, were described as idiots of 'not a bad type'.[110] Buckby could 'evidently understand most of what is said to him, but does not appear to have many words' and Robinson had 'learnt her letters but not numbers'.[111] It could be more than coincidental that those who were not the 'bad type' of idiot tended to be capable of some work. They could have been put to employment within the asylum and their productivity contributed to the running and maintenance of the institution.

Alongside intellectual capabilities the appearance of a child was key to diagnosing idiocy. It was essential that the child looked an idiot and, more importantly, for this to be recorded. When Dorothy Maud Humphrey, aged seven, was admitted to the Three Counties Asylum it was noted 'she has the appearance of a child that has been an idiot from birth'.[112] Similarly, James Lidstone, admitted to the Northamptonshire institution, aged just three, was 'manifestly an idiot from his general appearance'.[113] Also, George Griffin admitted to Colney Hatch was said to be 'idiotic in expression'.[114] By labelling the appearance of these children their conditions and place within the asylum were also characterised. Dorothy Humphrey was capable of some conversation, but was crippled and unable to walk. Her appearance of being idiotic led to her admission to the asylum. Appearance was a key factor in the admission process and was at times more important than the debilitating physical impairments that patients displayed.

Under the broad diagnosis of idiocy the five asylums confined a large number of children described as epileptic. The rhetorical register describing these patients was similar to those suffering harmless conditions, but with added reference to fits, seizures or convulsions. For example, Edith Brown at Prestwich, William Stanley at Birmingham, Thomas Eastsmith and Matilda Wood at Colney Hatch, Charles Charlwood and Florence Randall at Northampton, and George Pugh and May Inskip at Three Counties were all described as being unable to speak, incoherent, simple or lacking intelligence as well as epileptic.[115] An exception to this model of description was John Collyer, aged thirteen admitted to Colney Hatch in 1854; he could partake in intelligent conversation and had a 'worn aspect' that was not characteristic of idiocy, but he suffered from 'fits'.[116] While modern ideas of 'fits' and epilepsy are fixed through our understanding of the condition and representations in the media, during the nineteenth century the term was used frequently without effective explanation. Case notes often refer to 'fits' of excitement, passion, violence and screaming or more generally 'episodes' which could cloud judgement and confuse understanding of what exactly was being recorded. It is therefore worth considering that although 'fits' are mentioned generically they may be a value laden term and open to broader interpretation than epileptic seizures; for instance, children that suffered 'fits' when teething most likely did so because of high temperatures, rather than epilepsy. The Medical Officer at the Birmingham Union Workhouse succinctly explained that many epileptics 'were perfectly sane between the attacks, but during attacks were utterly uncertain'.[117] Due to the nature of epilepsy the Lunacy Acts made no provision for these cases and later in our period separate colonies were established to house this type of patient.

The situation was markedly different for those described as dangerous idiots or imbeciles. In these circumstances references to impaired intelligence or incoherence were replaced by statements detailing how the child was a danger either to themselves or those around them. Accessories such as knives, fires, stones, and windows featured regularly. Also the safety of younger siblings was often of paramount importance when framing the element of danger. For example, Thomas Woodcock, aged eight when admitted to Colney Hatch, was known to wake up in the night and wander around the house dragging his sister by the hair.[118] Although fewer in number than harmless or epileptic congenital patients, dangerous idiots still constituted a significant proportion of children admitted to the asylum.

Dangerous patients can be filtered into two further categories—those that were a danger unintentionally and those that were a danger vindictively. Alfred Ringrose, admitted to Colney Hatch, is an example of the former. His mother said he had no sense, he pulled cinders out of the fire and when they burnt his hands he dropped them on the floor.[119] Frederick Henson was prone to sleep walking and was also 'fond of the fire' at these times.[120] Patients of this type were rarer than those perceived to be vindictive or malicious.

'Restlessness' and 'excitability' were the key adjectives used to describe those admitted as violent and dangerous. These individuals were usually beyond the control of their parents or were difficult to manage in the workhouse.[121] For example, John Kersey, aged eight, admitted to Colney Hatch in 1869, was said by his mother to be uncontrollable during his violent fits.[122] Caroline Holsey, at the age of five was said to be 'restless ... and too dangerous for the children's ward' at Three Counties.[123] Ada Hands, aged ten, Birmingham, was difficult to control and unfit to be at home.[124] Frederick Farren threw chairs at Colney Hatch,[125] Charles Fisher was prone to get on the roofs of his neighbours' houses and knock their chimney pots down,[126] and Robert Harris tried to stab his mother with a knife.[127] William Lack at Northampton was said to cause trouble at home; he 'throws knives and forks at people and is dangerous about the fire'.[128] Charles Broughton, also confined at the Northamptonshire asylum, was said to be always 'punching or biting other children ... beyond control'.[129] Frederick Payne threatened another child with a knife and John Feltham destroyed three shirts in the workhouse.[130] These examples effectively demonstrate the threats of physical danger to others, especially children, posed by these individuals. Within these behavioural descriptions the destruction of property also runs as a subtext in defining the dangerous.[131] While the harmless idiot patient was confined for care, the dangerous was confined for regulation.

The element of dangerousness, however, is one that requires a greater degree of analysis. For example, the Medical Certificate for Emma Nightingale clearly stated she was dangerous, but her asylum case notes read the opposite. The second observation of her stated 'not so troublesome as might be expected'. This was not an isolated incident; later entries read 'this child is not much trouble' and 'well conducted for an idiot'.[132] It could have been that the therapeutic environment of the asylum provided an instant amelioration of her condition but this seems unlikely. The case of John Wenborn has been discussed in greater depth elsewhere, but he was confined because he was a particular danger to his sister. When in the asylum, however, he did not display dangerous tendencies and provided no trouble other than suffering frequent epileptic seizures.[133] The issue of dangerousness was open to exaggeration, or even abuse, in order to guarantee admission of a child to the asylum.

Admission versus Observation

The cases of Nightingale and Wenborn demonstrate that asylum observations did not always reflect the descriptions made on medical certificates prior to confinement. The process of certification represented two separate but official medical discourses, each with differing motives for identifying and monitoring the insane.[134] So far, analysis has concentrated on the admission of the child to the asylum and on the language used to describe their condition on arrival. It has utilised the information provided from Certificates of Insanity and the initial examination of the child at the asylum. The language of insanity used in asylum casebooks appears to have remained relatively stable, both chronologically and geographically, throughout the period. This suggests a common medical rhetorical register for insanity, which might lead modern observers to conclude that diagnosis took place in a uniform, consistent, and objective medical structure. Closer scrutiny of case records demonstrates that the illnesses and disabilities of children, often described in common linguistic terms, in fact differed greatly in the asylum, and at times the behaviours that were crucial to confirming the insanity of a child were not displayed in the asylum at all.

The case of William Gunn provides an example of such discrepancy. He was admitted to the asylum in Northamptonshire in 1889; a key feature of his medical certificate was that his mother said he was incapable of education. Thus arguments made about the use of family testimony in identifying and diagnosing child patients are reinforced. It also demonstrates awareness amongst poor parents of the growing role education played in the construction of child insanity. In this case, however, the family's statement was challenged by the Medical Superintendent at the point of admission to the asylum. The casefile reads: 'contrary to his mother's statement he knows the letters perfectly and can count upon his fingers up to 8 or 10'.[135] The asylum rejected what it thought was the inexpert Poor Law medical opinion and in this instance was keen to stamp their perceived professional expertise on patients. Similarly, James Richardson was admitted to the Three Counties Asylum in 1876. James Wright, the Poor Law Medical Officer, stated that Richardson had told him there was 'a spider spinning webs in his head' and consequently sent him to the asylum.[136] When he arrived at the asylum Richardson contradicted this statement and told the Superintendent that he was sent because he refused to attend school. The patient was discharged showing 'no evidence of insanity' after three weeks of observation.

Not all discrepancies in behavioural observations, however, were evident at the point of admittance. Alfred Sowter was admitted to Colney Hatch in 1897. According to the medical certificate he was 'of inferior mental development and deficient in moral sense'.[137] He was alleged to be frequently violent and had even attempted to poison his mother. One week after admission he was described as being 'well behaved' and 'fairly cheerful'.[138] The observations continued in this vein until the patient was discharged one month after being admitted. The cases of James Richardson and Alfred Sowter show that admission to the asylum was, sometimes, achieved by constructing a narrative that was thought to fit the expectation of insane behaviour as defined by the Poor Law Amendment Act in 1834. These narratives were developed outside of the asylum and were quickly exposed by, and removed from, the institution.

Often a label of mental illness or disability could mask other symptoms of deviance that were disturbing to Victorian sensibilities. These behaviours are recorded within the observational notes of the casefiles and provide an insight into attitudes towards children and insanity. Harriet Meadows was admitted to Northampton Asylum aged five in 1884. She was said to have been 'a healthy child until 2 years old. Since then it has been imbecile.' Once confined within the asylum the inappropriate sexual actions of the child were what caused concern, rather than her imbecility. Her casefile recorded in 1888 there is 'no change in this little idiot except that she is often noticed to be fingering about the genitals'. The labels of idiot and imbecile were again used interchangeably. Later entries continued, 'no reason why she should be in an asylum'. Her inappropriate sexual behaviour continued throughout 1889 and it was recorded in two separate entries that she 'often masturbates at night' and 'this girl still practices her bad habit'.[139]

Harriet Meadows was not the only child to be referred to in these deviant terms. Albert Stanley admitted to the Birmingham institution was identified as a masturbator prior to his admission.[140] William Moore, confined in Northamptonshire, was described as 'a great masturbator' and was subjected to preventative measures, such as blistering and restraining to rectify his habit.[141] Also, John Cable admitted to Colney Hatch was stated by a nurse 'to regularly expose his person and is guilty of dirty tricks'.[142] Similarly, Lilla Ward was admitted to Three Counties when her mother said she could not be let out of the house because she acted indecently, 'pulling up her clothes and exposing her person'.[143] The examples of Meadows, Moore, and Cable were all witnessed from inside the asylum and provide medical observations of such behaviour. It could be argued that Lilla Ward's mother was presenting a set of behaviours designed to provoke admission to an asylum rather than workhouse and consequently might be less reliable. These patients all, however, challenged Victorian social sensibilities and attitudes towards the appropriate behaviour of children both in private and in public. The historiography has not yet demonstrated that similar behaviours were considered unacceptable in the adult asylum population. The sexualised behaviour of the Victorian child can thus be seen as dangerous and asylum doctors were aware of the need for confinement and regulation.

The observational records of child patients make it possible to draw some judgements of how the asylum responded to the children who were confined within it. There is evidence to suggest that not only were children of limited value because of their incurable conditions but they were also dehumanised inside the asylum.[144] Harriet Meadows, mentioned above, was referred to as 'it' and a 'devil' within her case notes.[145] Albert Mitchell, aged thirteen when admitted to Berrywood, was stated to be worse than an animal in his file.[146] George Collett, confined in Colney Hatch, aged nine, was said to be more animal than human.[147] Alfred Brett also resident in Colney Hatch was more like 'one of the brute creations than a child'.[148] Oliver Frank Bailey at Northampton was said to be 'a repulsive looking idiot boy'.[149] William Morris was described as 'a puny, deformed child', and George Jelly 'a wretched little child'.[150] The attitudes directed towards these children were not always open and caring. It seems that the institution of care and respite looked down on these children and treated them, at times, with disdain.

Conclusion

The chapter has explored how child insanity was constructed across our five institutions during the nineteenth century. Child patients have been counted, the causes and nature of their illnesses and disabilities explored, and to some extent their asylum experiences have for the first time also been revealed. It is clear that child insanity was complex and varied both in lay and professional environment, but admissions and the language used to describe conditions was surprisingly uniform. Going forward it is important to bear in mind the similarities in diagnoses as we begin to consider the variation in treatment of these children. While the language used to describe child insanity remained consistent, methods of identifying the insane did evolve. The growth of compulsory schooling saw a shift from private, family based identification of mental impairment to a more public, state influenced process. Such fluidity in the medical discourse surrounding insanity in the nineteenth century, while to some extent noted by the literature, is evident. Next we must look to how the asylum was utilised at typological and regional levels. The quantitative discussions earlier in this chapter reveal that access to and confinement in the asylum was uneven across the five regions in focus and it is to this issue that we now turn.

Notes

1. M. Foucault, *Madness and Civilisation: A History of Insanity in the Age of Reason* (London: Routledge, reprint 2001) originally *Histoire de la folie á l'age classique* (1961), Chap 2; 48 Geo. III, c. 96.
2. J. Andrews and A. Scull, *Customers and Patrons of the Mad-Trade: The Management of Lunacy in Eighteenth-Century London* (London: University of California Press, 2003); W. Parry-Jones, *The Trade in Lunacy: A Study of the Private Madhouses in England in the Eighteenth and Nineteenth Centuries* (London: Routledge, 1972).
3. 55 Geo. III, c.46.
4. The first asylums built were in the counties of Bedfordshire, Cornwall, Gloucestershire, Lincoln, Norfolk, Nottinghamshire, Staffordshire, Suffolk, and two county asylums were built in the more densely populated counties of Yorkshire and Lancashire. L. Smith, *Cure, Comfort and Safe Custody: Pauper Lunatic Asylums in Early Nineteenth-Century England* (London: Leicester University Press, 1999), p. 82.
5. A. Digby, 'Changes in the Asylum: The Case of York, 1777–1815,' *The Economic History Review*, 36/2 (1983), pp. 218–239, p. 222. A. Suzuki, 'The Politics and Ideology of Non-Restraint: The Case of the Hanwell Asylum,' *Medical History*, 39 (1995), pp. 1–17.
6. Foucault, *Madness and Civilization.*
7. Smith, *Cure, Comfort and Safe Custody*, Chap. 6.
8. 8 & 9 Vict., c. 100.
9. P. McCandless, 'Liberty and Lunacy: The Victorians and Wrongful Confinement,' in A. Scull (ed.), *Madhouses, Mad-Doctors, and Madmen:*

The Social History of Psychiatry in the Victorian Era (London: Athlone, 1981), pp. 339–362.

10. R. Hunter and I. MacAlpine, *Psychiatry for the Poor: 1851 Colney Hatch Asylum—Friern Hospital 1973 A Medical and Social History* (London: Dawsons, 1974), p. 17; P. Bartlett, *The Poor Law of Lunacy: The Administration of Pauper Lunatics in Mid-Nineteenth-Century England* (London: Leicester University Press, 1999); P. Bartlett, 'The Asylum and the Poor Law: The Productive Alliance,' in J. Melling and B. Forsythe (eds.), *Insanity, Institutions and Society, 1800–1914: A Social History of Madness in Comparative Perspective* (Abingdon: Routledge), pp. 48–67, p. 51.
11. LMA, Friern Hospital (Colney Hatch), Male Casebook 9, H12/CH/B/13/009, George Hamilton, Admission no. 2970, p. 92.
12. Bartlett, *Poor Law of Lunacy*, pp. 102–103.
13. Ibid., p. 134.
14. V. Skultans, *English Madness: Ideas on Insanity, 1580–1890* (London: Routledge, 1979), p. 103.
15. Ibid.
16. J. Melling, R. Adair, and B. Forsythe, '"A Proper Lunatic for Two Years": Pauper Lunatic Children in Victorian and Edwardian England. Child Admissions to the Devon County Lunatic Asylum, 1845–1914,' *Journal of Social History*, 31/2 (1997), pp. 371–405.
17. P. Bartlett, *Poor Law of Lunacy*, p. 97.
18. 49 Vict. c. 25.
19. A. Wood Renton, *The Law and Practice in Lunacy: With the Lunacy Acts 1890–1 (consolidated and annotated): The Rules of the Lunacy Commissioners 1895: The Idiots Act 1886: The Vacating of Seats Act 1886* (London: Stevens & Haynes, 1896), p. 777.
20. Ibid., p. 784.
21. K. Jones, *Mental Health and Social Policy 1845–1959* (London: Routledge, 1960), p. 47.
22. Emphasis is my own. 54 Vict. c. 3.
23. These bodies were created by the Local Government Act of 1888.
24. K. Jones, *Mental Health and Social Policy*, p. 40.
25. K. Jones, *Asylums and After: A Revised History of the Mental Health Services: From the Early 18th Century to the Late 1990s* (London: Athlone, 1993), p. 120.
26. This distinction was posited by J. Haslam, *A Letter to the Lord Chancellor on the Nature and Interpretation of Unsoundness of Mind and Imbecility of Intellect* (London: R. Hunter, 1823); F. Winslow, *The Plea of Insanity in Criminal Cases* (London: H. Renshaw, 1843); E. Seguin, *Idiocy: And*

its Treatment by the Physiological Method (New York: Brandows, 1866, reprinted New York: Teachers College, Columbia University, 1907).

27. *Report of the Metropolitan Commissioners in Lunacy* (London: Bradbury and Evans, 1844).
28. A. Borsay, *Disability and Social Policy in Britain since 1750* (Basingstoke: Palgrave Macmillan, 2005), p. 39.
29. D. Wright, *Mental Disability in Victorian England: The Earlswood Asylum, 1847–1901* (Oxford: Clarendon, 2001), p. 82; Wright, 'Familial Care of "Idiot" Children in Victorian England,' in P. Horden and R. Smith (eds.), *The Locus of Care: Families, Communities, Institutions and the Provision of Welfare since Antiquity* (London: Routledge, 1997), pp. 176–197, p. 183; The role of healthy children as care providers for their younger siblings is discussed by J. Parr, *Labouring Children: British Immigrant Apprentices to Canada, 1869–1924* (London: Croom Helm, 1980), pp. 16–19.
30. S. G. Howe, 'On the Causes of Idiocy,' in M. Rosen, G. R. Clark, M.S. Kivitz (eds.), *The History of Mental Retardation, Collected Papers* (paper first published 1848, collection published Baltimore: University Park Press, 1976), pp. 34–37.
31. E. Seguin, *Idiocy: And its Treatment by the Physiological Method* (New York: Brandows, 1866 reprinted New York: Teachers College, Columbia University, 1907), p. 29; M.E. Talbot, *Edoward Seguin* (New York: Teacher's College Press, 1964); H. Lane, *The Wild Boy of Aveyron* (St Albans: Paladin, 1979), pp. 261–278.
32. See P. Bartlett, *Poor Law of Lunacy*, pp. 88–90.
33. Wright, *Earlswood*, p. 17.
34. K. Price, *A Regional, Quantitative and Qualitative Study of the Employment, Disciplining and Discharging of Workhouse Medical Officers of the New Poor Law throughout Nineteenth-Century England and Wales* (Oxford Brookes University: Unpublished PhD thesis 2008).
35. Melling et al., 'Proper Idiot'. p. 375.
36. H. Cunningham, *The Children of the Poor: Representations of Childhood since the Seventeenth Century* (Oxford: Blackwell, 1991); D. Wardle, *The Rise of the Schooled Society: The History of Formal Schooling in England* (London: Routledge, 1974).
37. Wright, '"Childlike in his Innocence": Lay Attitudes towards "Idiots" and "Imbeciles" in Victorian England,' in D. Wright and A. Digby (eds.), *From Idiocy to Mental Deficiency: Historical Perspectives on People with Learning Disabilities*, pp. 118–133, pp. 122–124.
38. NRO, St Crispin Collection, Out of County Casebook 2, NCLA/6/2/2/17, Amos Tullet, Admission no. 2734, p. 236.

39. NRO, St Crispin Collection, Male Casebook 9, NCLA/6/2/2/9, Alfred Hamp, Admission no. 4677, p. 31.
40. BLA, Three Counties, Female Casebook 3, LF29/3, Alice Popper, Admission no. 2589, p. 310.
41. Ibid., p. 130.
42. L. Ray, 'Models of Madness in Victorian Asylum Practice,' *European Journal of Sociology*, 22/2 (1981), pp. 229–264.
43. Ibid.
44. For accuracy the total number of patients used for this calculation is 753. This is due to a number of patients having casefiles that are not accessible due to loss or damage.
45. S.G. Howe, 'On the Causes of Idiocy,' p. 34.
46. Seguin, *Idiocy*, p. 31.
47. D.H. Tuke, *Insanity in Ancient and Modern Life with Chapters on its Prevention* (London: Macmillan, 1878).
48. NRO, St Crispin Collection, Out of County Casebook 1, NCLA6/2/2/16, Ellen Wilkins, Admission no. 2749, p. 366; LMA, Friern Hospital (Colney Hatch), Male Casebook 4, H12/CH/B/13/004, William Hammond, Admission no. 12298, p. 58; NRO, St Crispin Collection, Male Casebook 7, NCLA/6/2/2/7, Frederick Tilley, Admission no. 3950, p. 182.
49. xxx.
50. NRO, St Crispin Collection, Male Casebook 3, NCLA/6/2/2/3, Stephen Webster, Admission no. 1306, p. 205.
51. NRO, St Crispin Collection, Male Casebook 9, NCLA/6/2/2/9, William Brazier, Admission no. 4813, p. 77.
52. BLA, Three Counties, Male Casebook 7, LF31/7, Bertram Waring, Admission no. 4346, p. 80.
53. BLA, Three Counties, Male Casebook 3, LF31/3, Ernest Morgan, Admission no. 2554, p. 206; BLA, Three Counties, Female Casebook 15, LF29/15, Agnes Reeve, Admission no. 2194, p. 8399.
54. BCA, All Saints Asylum, Male Casebook 29, MS344/12/29, Samuel Gardiner, pp. 621–622; BCA, All Saints Asylum Female Casebook 46, MS344/12/46, Florry Wright, pp. 669–672.
55. BCA, All Saints Asylum, Male Casebook 11, MS344/12/11, George Avery, pp.69–70.
56. GMCRO, Prestwich, Female casebook, ADMF/2/2, Ann Kelly, admission no. 9341.
57. C. Smith, 'Living with Insanity: Narratives of Poverty, Pauperism and Sickness in Asylum Records 1840–1876,' in A. Gestrich, E. Hurren, and S. King (eds.), *Poverty and Sickness in Modern Europe: Narratives of the Sick Poor, 1780–1938* (London: Continuum, 2012), pp. 117–142.

58. Price, *Regional, Quantitative and Qualitative*, has suggested long-term patients could be considered a nuisance by medical men, p. 315; Also see A. Suzuki, "Enclosing and Disclosing Lunatics within the Family Walls: Domestic Psychiatric Regime and the Public Sphere in Early Nineteenth-Century England,' in Bartlett and Wright, *Outside the Walls of the Asylum: The History of Care in the Community 1750–2000* (London: Athlone, 1999), pp. 115–131.
59. Ray, 'Models of Madness,' p. 237.
60. British Library, London County Council, 'A review of the work of the council during the year ended 31st March, 1894 an address by Mr John Hutton, Chairman of the Council,' L.C.C. 108, p. 10.
61. F. Galton, *Hereditary Genius* (London: Macmillan, 1869); F. Galton, *Inquiries into Human Faculty and its Development* (London: J.M Dent & Company, 1883); M. Bulmer, *Francis Galton: Pioneer of Heredity and Biometry* (Baltimore: John Hopkins University Press, 2003).
62. Ibid., p. 369.
63. H. Maudsley, *Body and Mind* (London: Macmillan, 1873), p. 276; and *Responsibility in Mental Disease* (London: S. King & co., 1874).
64. 'Facts of Insanity' is a section of the casebooks used to record the symptoms of patients on their admission to the asylum. The section usually has space for both medical and lay observations.
65. A. Kleinman, *The Illness Narratives: Suffering, Healing and the Human Condition* (New York: Basic Books, 1988), pp. 3–5.
66. Wright 'Childlike'; Melling et al., 'Proper Lunatic,' p. 377.
67. BLA, Three Counties, Male Casebook 4, LF31/4, George Canfield, Admission no. 2949, p. 92.
68. LMA, Friern Hospital Colney Hatch, Male Casebook 46, H12/CH/B/13/046, Sydney Virtue, ad no. 12863, p. 25.
69. Wright, 'Childlike'.
70. A. Scull, *Museums of Madness: The Social Organization of Insanity in Nineteenth-Century England* (London: Allen Lane, 1979); Scull, *The Most Solitary of Afflictions: Madness and Society in Britain 1700–1900* (London: Yale University Press, 1993).
71. Wright, *Earlswood*; Wright, 'Getting Out of the Asylum: Understanding the Confinement of the Insane in the Nineteenth Century,' *Social History of Medicine*, 10/1, pp. 137–155.; C. Smith, 'Living with Insanity,' p. 119.
72. Wright, *Earlswood*, p. 82; R. Smith, 'Some Issues Concerning Families and their Property in Rural England, 1250–1800,' in Smith (ed.), *Land, Kinship and Life-Cycle* (Cambridge: Cambridge University Press, 1985), pp. 1–86, pp. 68–69; Parr, *Labouring Children*, Chap. 1.

73. Scull, Museums; C. Smith, 'Family, Community and the Victorian Asylum: A Case Study of Northampton General Lunatic Asylum and its Pauper Lunatics,' *Family and Community History*, 9/2, pp. 109–124.
74. Phthisis was often used interchangeably with other terms such as consumption and tuberculosis.
75. This view was first put forward by the noted Edinburgh psychiatrist, and from 1898 President of the Child Study Association, Thomas Clouston and is examined in depth by G. E Berrios, 'Phthisical Insanity,' *History of Psychiatry*, 16/4 (2005), pp. 473–495.
76. NRO, St Crispin Collection, Male Casebook 8, NCLA/6/2/2/8, John Scott, Admission no. 4193, p. 39.
77. BCA, All Saints, Male Casebook 13, MS344/12/13, Tom Skirrow, Admission no. 8621, pp. 429–430.
78. Again this figure is most likely more than the 103 stated. There are 104 cases that have unknown causes of death. These are mainly due to data protection embargos and case notes being recorded in continuation books that have been lost or are not fit for public viewing. The second largest cause of death was epilepsy which accounted for 63 deaths within the sample.
79. C. Smith, 'Living with Insanity'.
80. NRO, St Crispin Collection, Male Casebook 9, NCLA/6/2/2/9, Walter Quinnell, Admission no. 4863, p. 108.
81. NRO, St Crispin Collection, Male Casebook 8, NCLA/6/2/2/8, Sidney Carrington, Admission no. 4501, p. 188.
82. LMA, Friern Hospital (Colney Hatch), Female Casebook 33, H12/CH/B/11/033, Henrietta Lamb, Admission no. 11047, p. 192.
83. Percentage breakdown by institution of admissions of idiots and imbeciles; Birmingham 52 %, Colney Hatch 71 %, Manchester 61 %, Northampton 93 %, Three Counties 74 %. Issues of regional difference will be explored in Chap. 5.
84. G. Grabham, *BMJ*, 16 January 1875, p. 74.
85. G. E. Shuttleworth, *BMJ*, 30 January 1886, pp. 183–186.
86. M. Jackson, 'Institutional Provision for the Feeble-Minded in Edwardian England: Sandlebridge and the Scientific Morality of Permanent Care,' in D. Wright and A. Digby (eds.), *From Idiocy to Mental Deficiency: Historical Perspectives on People with Learning Disabilities* (London: Routledge, 1996), pp. 161–183.
87. M. K. Simpson, 'Othering Intellectual Disability: Two Models of Classification from the Nineteenth Century,' *Theory Psychology*, 22/5 (2012), pp. 541–556.
88. A. Borsay, *Disability and Social Policy*, p. 71.

89. D. Wright, 'Learning Disability and the New Poor Law in England, 1834–1867,' *Disability and Society*, 15/5 (2000), pp. 731–745, p. 742.
90. Ibid.; also see C. Cox and H. Marland, '"A Burden on the County": Madness, Institutions of Confinement and the Irish Patient in Victorian Lancashire,' *Social History of Medicine*, 28/2 (2015), pp. 263–287.
91. LMA, Friern Hospital (Colney Hatch), Male Casebook 2, H12/CH/B/13/002, John Harvey, Admission no. 628, p. 82.
92. BLA, Three Counties, Female Casebook 1, LF29/1, Sarah Ann Goodman, Admission no. 340, p. 121.
93. NRO, St Crispin Collection, Female Casebook 5, NCLA6/2/1/5, Mabel Adkins, Admission no. 2403, p. 228.
94. Wellcome Library, G.E. Shuttleworth, 'On the Treatment of Children Mentally Deficient. An Address to the Union of Teachers of the Deaf and Dumb on the Pure Oral System,' (1895), MS. 4579, p. 10.
95. LRO, Prestwich, Male Casebook 1, QAM6/6/1, Edward Ridings, Admission no. 68.
96. BLA, Three Counties, Female Casebook 20, LF29/20, Jane Denifer, Admission no. 10295, p. 8.
97. BLA, Three Counties, Female Casebook 19, LF29/19, Eliza Perry, Admission no. 9852, p. 16.
98. NRO, St Crispin Collection, Male Casebook 5, NCLA/6/2/2/5, Arthur Harry White, Admission no. 2427, p. 141.
99. BLA, Three Counties, Female Casebook 15, LF29/15, Constance May Watson, Admission no. 8100, p. 94.
100. NRO, St Crispin Collection, Out of County Casebook 2, NCLA/6/2/3/2, John McCormack, Admission no. 3095, p. 378.
101. NRO, St Crispin Collection, Male Casebook 5, NCLA/6/2/2/5, John Tanner, p. 51, was asked and knew the days of the week; NRO, St Crispin Collection, Male Casebook 5, NCLA/6/2/2/5, Sidney Bishop, p. 96 knew his family and the days of the week.
102. LRO, Prestwich, Male Casebook 32, QAM6/6/32, Jacob Gaffey, Admission no. 7628, did not know the names of his family members.
103. LMA, Friern Hospital (Colney Hatch), Louisa Barley (Female Casebook 1a, H12/CH/B/11/001a, Admission no. 923), Rhoda Key (Admission Register 6, H12/CH/B/01/006, Admission no. 4189), and Frederick Lawrence (Male Casebook 2, H12/CH/B/13/002, Admission no. 687) were all judged on their ability to read and write.
104. NRO, St Crispin Collection, Male Casebook 5, NCLA/6/2/2/5, Ernest Cross, Admission no. 2404, p. 134.
105. NRO, St Crispin Collection, Male Casebook 4, NCLA/6/2/2/4, Joseph Albert Harris, Admission no. 1550, p. 190.
106. NRO, Sidney Bishop, p. 96.

107. NRO, St Crispin Collection, Female Casebook 7, NCLA/6/2/1/7, Ellen Tarry, Admission no. 3167, p. 6.
108. BLA, Three Counties, Female Casebook 3, LF29/3, Alice Popper, Admission no. 2589, p. 310.
109. W.A.F. Browne, 'What Asylums Were, Are, and Ought to be,' 1837, in A. Scull (ed.), *The Asylum as Utopia: W.A.F. Browne and the Mid-Nineteenth Century Consolidation of Psychiatry* (London: Routledge, 1991), pp. 7–8.
110. NRO, St Crispin Collection, Female Casebook 6, NCLA/6/2/1/6, Annie Clarke, Admission no. 2720, p. 89; Male Patient Casebook 6, NCLA/6/2/2/6, George Buckby, Admission no. 3390, p. 211; Out of County Casebook 1, NCLA/6/2/3/1, Kate Robinson, Admission no. 2726, p. 358.
111. NRO, George Buckby, p. 211.
112. BLA, Three Counties, Female Casebook 18, LF29/18, Dorothy Maud Humphrey, Admission no. 9773, p. 218.
113. NRO, St Crispin Collection, Out of County CaseBook 2, NCLA/6/2/3/1, James Lidstone, ad no. 2529, p. 174.
114. LMA, Friern Hospital (Colney Hatch), Male Casebook 11, H12/CH/B/13/011, George Griffin, Admission no. 3744.
115. LRO, Prestwich, Female Casebook 25, QAM6/5/25, Edith Brown, Admission no. 6436; BCA, All Saints, Male Casebook 4, MS344/12/4, William Stanley, Admission no. 5219; LMA, Friern Hospital (Colney Hatch), Male Casebook 20, H12/CH/B/13/020, Thomas Eastsmith, Admission no. 5268; LMA Friern Hospital (Colney Hatch), Female Casebook 1b, H12/CH/B/11/001b, Matilda Wood, Admission no. 960; NRO, St Crispin Collection, Out of County Casebook 2, NCLA/6/2/3/2, Charles Charlwood, Admission no. 2413, p. 134; NRO, St Crispin Collection, Female Casebook 10, NCLA/6/2/1/10, Florence Randall, Admission no. 5019, p. 45; BLA, Three Counties, Male Casebook 5, LF31/5, George Pugh, Admission no. 3285, p. 58; BLA, Three Counties, Female Casebook 17, LF29/17, May Inskip, Admission no. 9305, p. 230.
116. LMA, Friern Hospital (Colney Hatch), Male Casebook 2, H12/CH/B/13/002, John Collyer, Admission no. 1029.
117. BCA, Birmingham Union Infirmary Sub-Committee 1882–1883, GP/B/2/4/1/1, 3 November 1882.
118. LMA, Friern Hospital (Colney Hatch), Male Casebook 15, H12/CH/B/13/015, Thomas Woodcock, Admission no. 4441.
119. LMA, Friern Hospital (Colney Hatch), Male Casebook 23, H12/CH/B/13/023, Alfred Ringrose, Admission no. 6218.

120. NRO, St Crispin Collection, Male Casebook 5, NCLA/6/2/2/5, Frederick Henson, Admission no. 2650, p. 190.
121. Borsay, *Disability and Social Policy*, p. 71; Wright, 'Learning Disability and the Poor Law,' p. 742.
122. LMA, Friern Hospital (Colney Hatch), Male Casebook 15, H12/CH/B/13/015, John Kersey, Admission no. 4421.
123. BLA, Three Counties, Female Casebook 3, LF29/3, Caroline Holsey, Admission no. 2194, p. 97.
124. BCA, All Saints, Female Casebook 19, MS344/12/61, Ada Hands, pp. 501–503.
125. LMA, Friern Hospital (Colney Hatch), Male Casebook 29, H12/CH/B/13/029, Frederick Farren, Admission no. 7763.
126. LMA, Friern Hospital (Colney Hatch), Male Casebook 32, H12/CH/B/13/032, Charles Fisher, Admission no. 8734, p. 110.
127. LMA, Friern Hospital (Colney Hatch), Male Casebook 28, H12/CH/B/13/02/, Robert Harris, Admission no. 7525.
128. NRO, St Crispin Collection, Male Casebook 4, NCLA/6/2/2/4, William Lack, Admission no. 1713, p. 95.
129. NRO, St Crispin Collection, Male Casebook 5, NCLA/6/2/2/5, Charles Broughton, Admission no. 2535, p. 173.
130. NRO, St Crispin Collection, Male Casebook 11, NCLA/6/2/2/11, Frederick Payne, Admission no. 5820, p. 168; LMA, Friern Hospital (Colney Hatch), Male Casebook 33, H12/CH/B/13/033, John Feltham, Admission no. 9052, p. 140.
131. L. Smith, 'Your Very Thankful Inmate: Discovering the Patients of an early County Lunatic Asylum,' *Social History of Medicine*, 21 (2008), pp. 237–252.
132. NRO, St Crispin Collection, Female Casebook 3, NCLA/6/2/1/3, Emma Nightingale, Admission no. 1318, p. 232.
133. S.J. Taylor, '"All His Ways are Those of an Idiot:" The Admission, Treatment of and Social reaction to Two Idiot Children of Northampton Pauper Lunatic Asylum,' *Family and Community History*, 15/1, pp. 34–43.
134. Bartlett, *Poor Law of Lunacy*.
135. NRO, St Crispin Collection, Male Casebook 5, NCLA/6/2/2/5, William Gunn, Admission no. 2439, p. 146.
136. BLA, Three Counties, Male Casebook 4, LF31/4, James Richardson, Admission no. 2898, p. 71.
137. LMA, Friern Hospital (Colney Hatch), Male Casebook 44, H12/CH/B/13/044, Alfred Sowter, Admission no. 12634, p. 95.
138. Ibid., 20 February 1897, p. 95.
139. NRO, St Crispin Collection, Female Casebook 4, NCLA/6/2/1/4, Harriet Meadows, Admission no. 1719, p. 175.

140. BCA, All Saints, Male Casebook 14, MS344/12/14, Albert Stanley, Admission no. 9044, pp. 523–525.
141. NRO, St Crispin Collection, Out of County Casebook 2, NCLA/6/2/3/2, William Moore, Admission no. 2580, p. 202.
142. LMA Friern Hospital (Colney Hatch), Male Casebook 12, H12/CH/B/13/0012, John Cable, Admission no. 4027.
143. BLA, Three Counties, Female Casebook 15, LF29/15, Lilla Ward, Admission no. 8273, p. 172.
144. Wright, 'Learning Disability and New Poor law'.
145. NRO, Female Casebook, Meadows.
146. NRO, St Crispin Collection, Male Casebook 11, NCLA/6/2/2/11, Albert Mitchell, Admission no. 5623, p. 70.
147. LMA, Friern Hospital (Colney Hatch), Male Casebook 9, H12/CH/B/13/009, George Collett, Admission no. 3225, p. 348.
148. LMA, Friern Hospital (Colney Hatch), Male Casebook 12, H12/CH/B/13/012, Alfred Brett, Admission no. 3974.
149. NRO, St Crispin Collection, Male Casebook 9, NCLA/6/2/2/9, Oliver Bailey, Admission no. 5014, p. 188.
150. LMA, Friern Hospital (Colney Hatch), Male Casebook 8, H12/CH/B/13/008, William Morris, Admission no. 2474, p. 75; NRO, St Crispin Collection, Male Casebook 10, NCLA/6/2/2/10, George Jelly, Admission no. 5303, p. 121.

CHAPTER 3

Networks of Care: Asylum Children, Typology, and Experience

Did children receive the same care and treatment in each of the five asylums? For that matter, was there a standardised level of care across patient populations in the network of publicly funded asylums that stretched across England? These questions are particularly difficult to answer, primarily because the variations that occurred in admission, provision, and care between institutions has been a topic neglected by the literature.[1] By examining child patients and their lived experiences it is possible to evaluate sentiments towards the vulnerable (both physically and mentally) and the treatment that they received inside the asylum. This chapter compares their demographic profiles (age, gender, morbidity patterns), as well as geography (rural and urban origins), alongside the durations of their confinement. Such an approach complements established scholarship dealing with ethnicity, for example the Irish communities of Lancashire where experiences of migration often led to a breakdown of traditional family structures making young children more vulnerable to diseases of poverty.[2] Across the Pennines in Yorkshire and in the heartland of the Midlands, historians have likewise explored how the county asylum structure impacted on those labelled as insane living in overcrowded industrial and semi-industrial towns who were sent to either public or privately run institutions.[3] What all of these receptacles of the impaired and vulnerable had in common, however, was that their approaches towards child insanity were important parts of a larger mosaic of care that made up a very diverse private and publically run welfare sector. It was not then a 'total system'

S.J. Taylor, *Child Insanity in England, 1845-1907*, Palgrave Studies in the History of Childhood, DOI 10.1007/978-1-137-60027-1_3

as some scholars have assumed, but instead it offered diverse standards of treatment and practice in a spectrum of care options.[4]

In order to navigate this network of care it is essential to conduct a historical assessment of the key differences between the five representative institutions in the admission and treatment of children. A direct comparison of the urban Manchester and rural Northamptonshire asylums, by way of example, reveals the extreme variations that occurred. Following this the focus moves to the broader socio-economic environment that affected the treatment of the insane by assessing the impact of issues such as the Poor Law, migration, family structure, industrialisation, and urbanisation on the operation of the asylum for children living at the margins of society. The asylums are examined in terms of their demographic and geographic typologies so that any systematic patterns of care can be identified. This leads into a detailed historical discussion of the number of children admitted to each asylum, when admissions occurred, medical diagnoses, lengths of confinements, and how children departed institutions. The findings provide a thorough understanding of the children admitted and highlight the need for a comparative approach in order to fully understand asylum populations in the nineteenth century.

The Rural/Urban Divide

The differing nature of provision for children in rural and urban asylums can be identified through the practices of two institutions, and assessed, more uniquely, by looking at the broader regional socio-economic structure in which they existed. An examination of the Berrywood and Prestwich Asylums provides a clear and better understanding of institutional approaches and the differing attitudes towards the pauper insane that existed. The Berrywood Asylum of Northamptonshire opened in 1876, significantly later than the other institutions. Much like the Poor Law unions in the county the asylum was very much focused on minimising cost.[5] In fact, Berrywood's money-saving ethos helps to explain the significant number of children that it admitted. At first glance it might be assumed that such a parsimonious attitude would have restricted the number of youngsters that it received. Especially considering that asylum care was significantly more expensive than confinement in a workhouse. Yet from Fig. 3.1 it can be observed that Northamptonshire experienced a consistent flow of children to the asylum from both inside and outside of the county. This was not an uncommon experience. Poor Law Guardians

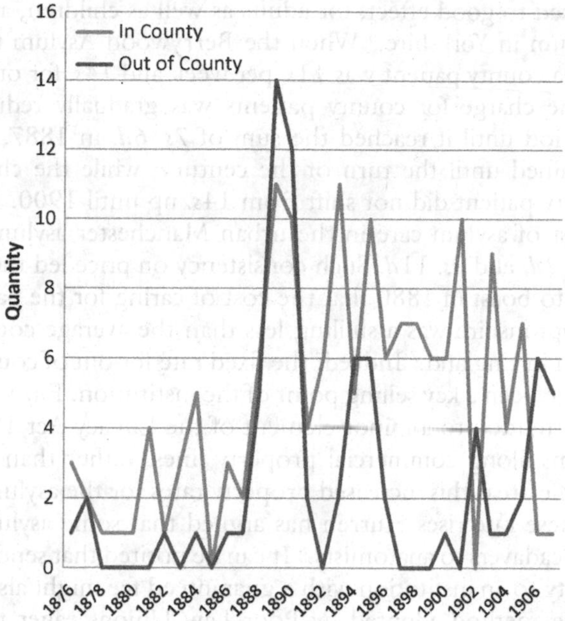

Fig. 3.1 County and out of county admissions to the Berrywood Asylum. *Source*: NRO, Male Patient Casebooks, NCLA/6/2/2/1-12; NRO Female Patient Casebooks, NCLA/6/2/1/1-13; Out of County Patient Casebooks, NCLA/6/2/3/1-2

regularly accessed the facilities of neighbouring counties, usually at a premium, when they were unable to admit lunatics to their local asylum. In total there were 61 out of county children admitted to Berrywood equating to 27 % of total child admissions. While on the face of it this might not appear a huge proportion, in comparison with the other four asylums there is a distinct difference in policy. At the Birmingham Asylum there were just three patients admitted from outside of the city, Colney Hatch admitted just four from beyond the metropolitan area, Manchester did not admit any patients from outside of its catchment area, and Three Counties confined five out of county patients.

The strategy of the Northamptonshire institution to admit patients from outside of the county, charged at a higher rate than local, was deliberate and served to reduce the cost for local ratepayers as well as providing a considerable source of profit to the asylum. Such a policy had also been used to good effect, for adults as well as children, at the North Riding Asylum in Yorkshire.[6] When the Berrywood Asylum first opened the cost for a county patient was 11*s.* per week and 14*s.* for out of county patients. The charge for county patients was gradually reduced over a ten-year period until it reached the sum of 7*s.* 6*d.* in 1887, an amount that it remained until the turn of the century; while the charge for an out of county patient did not shift from 14*s.* up until 1900. In comparison, the cost of asylum care in the urban Manchester asylum fluctuated between 8*s.* 2*d.* and 9*s.* 11*d.* Such consistency on price led those running Berrywood to boast in 1880 that the cost of caring for the pauper insane in Northamptonshire was a shilling less than the average county or borough asylum in England.[7] Indeed, the fixed rate for out of county patients may also have been a key selling point of the institution. Elizabeth Hurren has drawn attention to a minor element of the Lunacy Act 1890 that re-rated asylums along commercial property lines, rather than agricultural ones. In some areas this increased property rates for the asylum four-fold. To offset these rate rises Hurren has argued that some asylums covertly sold lunatic cadavers to anatomists.[8] It can be posited that sending patients out of county to an institution with a guaranteed fee might also have been a cost-saving method adopted by Poor Law Unions eager to avoid the fluctuating fees of their local asylums.

Asylum fees were not reduced for youngsters, so it is important to go further and highlight how children in Northamptonshire were seen as a specific vehicle for generating asylum profits. In 1888, the Berrywood institution opened an extension to the asylum that catered specifically for the needs of children. The 'children's block' was funded from the profits raised from out of county and private patients resident in the main buildings. Berrywood was very proud of its self-sufficiency and from its profits was also able to fund a hospital for infectious diseases, dining rooms for each ward, extended farm buildings, a reservoir, and a steam fire engine. A direct consequence of the new children's block was a peak in the number of out of county children admitted to the institution, evident in Fig. 3.1 above. It might be expected that the asylum was developing a specialism in the care of children, but it stated that the motive behind the block was to continue developing its own profitability by acting as a receptacle for children certified as insane. The asylum's annual report in 1888 declared:

> Advantage will be taken of the spare beds in this block to receive Idiot Children, either private or pauper, from other Counties. There are already

> six such cases, and the Visitors are about to enter into a contract with the Visitors of the Surrey County Asylum, at Cane Hill, for the reception of ten children. It may therefore be reasonably predicted that this addition to Berry Wood will prove not only beneficial to the unfortunate children but also a source of profit to the County.[9]

It is striking that the spare beds were earmarked for either private or out of county pauper patients and not insane children from the locality of the asylum. The large proportion of child patients can thus be a consequence of the institution's entrepreneurial attitude and its desire to maintain the position of being, by 1895, 'perhaps the only one [asylum] in England which has not drawn on the County for any Building or Repairs for seventeen years'.[10] The drive for profits was not as evident in the other four institutions and Northamptonshire's core values of independence, profitability, and sustainability are essential to explaining why it admitted such a large number of children.

Of course, in any discussion of asylum expansion and profits, it is vital to consider expenditure as well as income. The extant documents reveal limited information about staffing levels at the institution. The period 1891–1904 is missing from the records, but the asylum experienced most of its expansion during the 1880s. It is clear that the established drive for profitability was detrimental to the care of patients confined in the institution. In 1884, Berrywood housed 673 patients; by 1891 this figure had increased by about 20 % to 851. Over the same period the number of staff employed in positions of direct care, such as nurses and attendants, increased by just three, from 68 to 71 (5%). By 1891, only two of these were recorded as being directly employed to care for children in the asylum.[11] Consequently, a significant number of child deaths were recorded. These were most often from conditions unrelated to their mental health and might be explained by an element of neglect in their care caused by understaffing.

In Manchester an asymmetric approach to child admissions was taken. The Prestwich asylum did not proactively seek child patients, but much like at Berrywood the growth and development of this institution was instrumental to shaping its attitude towards them. Admissions to Prestwich are plotted in Fig. 3.2 and it can be seen that children entered in a stuttering fashion. There was a flurry of admissions following the opening of the asylum in 1851, but then children were not received until the 1860s. Much like in Northamptonshire, the increase in admissions from 1862 coin-

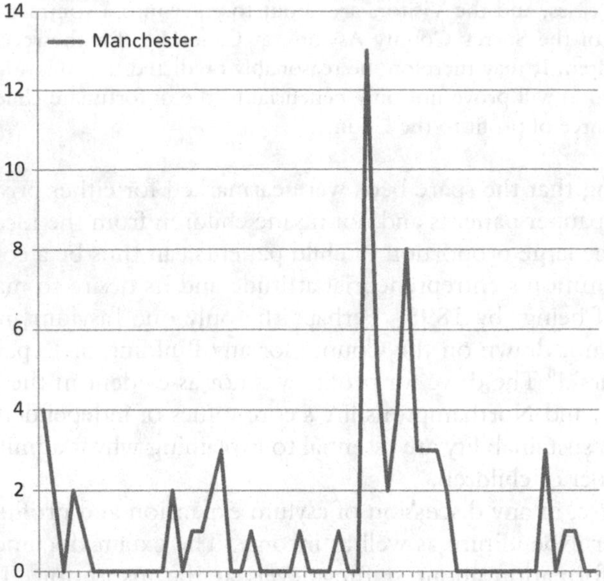

Fig. 3.2 Admissions to the Prestwich Asylum. *Source*: GMCRO, Male Patient Casebooks, ADMM/2/1-16; GMCRO, ADMF/2/1-21; LRO, Male Patient Casebooks, QAM/6/6/1-34; LRO, Female Patient Casebooks, QAM/6/6/1-34

cided with the opening of an extension to the asylum's facilities and an increase in capacity. Children were then admitted sporadically during the 1870s and early 1880s before the most intensive period of confining child patients occurred between the years 1884–1890. This spike in admissions, again like in Northamptonshire, was triggered by a significant expansion of the institution's facilities. In 1884 'The Annex' was opened to house 1100 chronic and harmless patients, thus making a considerable amount of space available for new cases.[12] The admission of children to Prestwich was not based on profitability or medical opinion, but rather the availability of new space in a recently extended institution.

'The Annex' was soon filled and it again became difficult to admit children to the Prestwich Asylum by 1890. Frustration at the situation was expressed in the correspondence sent from local Poor Law unions to the

Lancashire Asylums Board (LAB). In the February of 1895 a deputation of guardians from the West Derby Poor Law Union, 'supported by members of most of the Unions in the county', visited the LAB to discuss 'provision of special accommodation for young persons and children of weak intellect'.[13] It prompted the Ulverston Union Guardians to also complain that:

> the present practice of confining them [imbeciles and harmless lunatics], either in separate wards or allowing them to associate with sane persons in workhouses, is most undesirable, and in many respects highly objectionable; especially in the case of children of weak intellect associating with those who are not so afflicted.[14]

The inability to find space in the asylum for children was not due to the unsuitability of their conditions, but because asylums and workhouses in the region were stretched to breaking point. By August 1895 the West Derby Union, in frustration at being unable to transfer lunatics to the over-populated asylums of the county, announced that 'owing to the overcrowded state of Mill Road Infirmary, they will be unable to admit anymore lunatics'.[15] A rather dramatic step considering the size of the workhouse and reliance on it by agencies such as the police for depositing the pauper insane. In the meantime, the Ormskirk Union complained 'of the difficulties experienced by Guardians generally in finding accommodation for Lunatics'.[16] The pressure on space in the Lancashire asylum network was the most important factor in defining how children were dealt with throughout the period.

Underlining Difference—The Wider Picture

The management of children in and through asylums can only be understood by examining the approaches and practices of institutions. Before moving to the 'types' of children confined in each institution, it is worth shifting focus, briefly, to outside of the asylum walls and investigating the broader regional factors that affected admissions. It has already been demonstrated that the parsimonious nature of public institutions in Northamptonshire influenced the operation of the asylum, but there were also important social forces at work, such as industrialisation and urbanisation that affected the nature of care and confinement. The uneven pace of population growth in England and Wales has long been acknowledged.[17]

A key element of this irregular development was the sustained nature of expansion in manufacturing or commercial regions apposed with rural areas during the late eighteenth and nineteenth centuries. Tony Wrigley has shown that between the years 1811 and 1851 the population of England increased by 77 %, with a 49 % rise in the rural population and a non-rural population increase of 88 %. In the following forty years (1851–1891) the rural population grew by only 12 % while the non-rural underwent an expansion of 78 %, and the country as a whole 62 %.[18]

The population shift from rural to industrial was driven by a change in employment opportunities. By the end of the nineteenth century the proportion of the population employed in the agricultural sector in England was less than 10 %.[19] The rapid growth and expansion of new towns and cities was mirrored by relatively slow development in established market, cathedral or county towns.[20] Such experience is borne out by the regions examined here. The manufacturing centres of the West Midlands, such as Birmingham, grew much quicker and earlier than the established traditional county, cathedral, and market towns of rural areas, such as Northampton, Peterborough, and St Albans.[21] In Manchester the population grew rapidly from the 1750s with the period of peak expansion ending by 1831 and then growth slowing from that point.[22] In comparison, it has been argued that areas such as the East Midlands, of which Northamptonshire was a part, lacked a regional identity and unity that was present in industrial areas.[23] Child insanity thus needs to be located within a regional and social context that saw at 'least 75 per cent of late Victorian Britain's population made up of the urban industrial working class and their children'.[24] Admissions in the areas surrounding the Northamptonshire and Three Counties Asylums occurred during a time of development that resulted in significant shifts in the distributions of rural catchment populations.

The question of how population movement and growth affected the admission of insane pauper children to asylums as late as the second-half of the nineteenth century is particular poignant. Andrew Scull has provided an answer to this question, but he focused on the importance of industrialisation and urbanisation in pushing the insane towards the asylum.[25] It is clear, though, that industrial and urban asylums did not confine large numbers of children. Therefore we must find an explanation for why rural asylums more commonly confined mentally impaired or ill children, and at the heart of the matter are more specific catalysts of mobility and migration. The net population loss from the countryside to town was accelerated by a series of agricultural crises that struck the English countryside in the late nineteenth century. Wrigley has suggested that agriculture located near large centres of population and industry actually flourished during the mid-nineteenth century, rather than retarding growth by drawing in agricultural labourers to urban centres with offers of higher wages.[26] The rural regions examined here were therefore more likely to have experienced stagnation due to their distance from industrial centres. Alongside these developments the relationship between agricultural downturn and insanity had been well established contemporaneously. An increase in patient admissions to Yorkshire's East Riding Asylum during 1881 was attributed to 'the distress which has been widely and severely felt, but quietly borne, in the purely agricultural district from which the population of the asylum is drawn'.[27] However, how such times of economic depression impacted on children, rather than adults, is not as well understood.

The years 1876–1878, 1879–1884, and 1893–1896 were all particularly damaging in the rural regions of the east and south of England. These agricultural crises had a profound impact on the experience of Northamptonshire specifically. A consequence of downturn saw unskilled agricultural labourers migrating to the towns of Northampton, Kettering, Wellingborough, and Rushden. The historiography has suggested that these workers remained in the county rather than moving to industrial areas that were further afield. John Stobart stated that workers tended to remain near to home and there was no evidence of widespread migration from the East Midlands to the West Midlands and the north.[28] More generally, it has been demonstrated that throughout the nineteenth century people were tied to their locality and the mean distance migrated was just 32 km, with three-quarters of migrants travelling less than 20 km.[29] Within this population movement only 12.4 % of migrants travelled alone, meaning that children were an important part of population movement. Northamptonshire's towns were consequently forced to absorb an excess of labour.

In Manchester with the surrounding textile trade and the multiple opportunities connected to the metal works of Birmingham and its associated areas it would have been possible to accommodate such a migration of unskilled workers. The primary trade in Northamptonshire was the production of boots and shoes, an industry that by 1851 employed 13,254 people in the county, equivalent to 6 % of the population.[30] The majority of these were based in a domestic setting and while the 1850s witnessed the coming of the first factories for shoe making, production largely remained outside of factories until the mid 1890s by which time over 40,000 people were employed in some 400 factories.[31] As agriculture slumped during the 1870s, the boot and shoe trade boomed. It was spurred on by large orders from the French Government for army boots during the Franco-Prussian war. The combination of industrial boom and agricultural decline created a set of circumstances that accelerated the flood of workers to Northamptonshire's towns and consequently the surplus of labour meant that wages were kept at extremely low levels. Northampton's Methodist Minister, Revd G. Harrison, complained that the deprived nature of the towns in the county was caused by the 'ruinous competition amongst manufacturers [that] had reduced wages at every point until instead of being fair labour it was complete slavery'.[32] Towards the end of the nineteenth century, this situation was brought to the fore when a Royal Commission looking into labour migration was appointed. It stated 'that one question which will be strongly pressed on the attention of the Labour Commission is the migration of labourers from the country districts to the large towns … this is regarded as a serious matter, on account of its effect upon wages and the advantage which it gives to the employers in the case of a strike'.[33] The increased number of people in these towns consequently led to more families facing economic crisis and requesting assistance from the Poor Law.

Agricultural workers in Northamptonshire had been accustomed to undertaking some work, often domestically, in the boot and shoe trade to supplement their incomes, but this was not the case for agricultural workers in the other rural counties considered here. The areas surrounding the Three Counties Asylum faced different problems. While most migration undertaken by agricultural workers was relatively modest it does not mean there was not pressure to move further afield. The *Bucks Herald* reported in 1873 that 'men who are attached to their native homes—to the homes of their fathers—[were] migrating under pressure to the north of England, to engage in a class of work wholly unsuited to their inclinations, and to their constitutions'.[34] The supposed pressure was the promise of higher wages. The previous November the *Herald* had stated that the agricultural labourer 'has lived all his life upon the farm; he has been trained to habits which make him unsuitable to migrate to manufacturing districts where wages are higher'.[35] It is clear that the industrial north was considered an unsuitable destination for the rural population. The *Bucks Herald* paternalistically announced that if you 'take the agricultural labourer away from the dull monotony of life in the south of England, and set him down amid the whirl and hissing sound of factory life … he will be bewildered and amazed'.[36] The transition from rural to urban life was more difficult than is often perceived. There were contemporary concerns about urbanisation and it is important to bear in mind that those in agricultural areas were not easily lured to towns and cities.

During the period 1851–1901 the population of Kettering in Northamptonshire increased from 5000 to almost 30,000 and Rushden from 1460 to 12,453.[37] The boot and shoe trade could not adapt to cater for the flood of agricultural workers who lacked the skills to undertake the limited factory work available. Consequently, welfare provision was stretched to breaking point and social crisis ensued. But such a situation was not just an issue for the large towns, there were also consequences for some of the villages in the county. For example, the communities of Hackleton and Piddington, to the south of Northampton, experienced expansion through the building of shoe and boot factories in close proximity. In these locations the 'migration of the young people of the villages to the town has almost entirely stopped'.[38] The villages had become accustomed to losing its population to larger towns and experienced population growth due to the success of local industry. Those that chose to remain due to the boom were 'met by a very grave difficulty—that of a house in which to live. Not one can be got for love or money.'[39] Subsequently, the experience of Northamptonshire's industrialisation resulted in social crises, whether in towns or villages. The limited employment opportunities are a partial explanation for why so many children found their way to the asylum. Those with mental impairments would have been a drain on the family economy in terms of time and money and at an even greater disadvantage when they entered the labour market in comparison with their able-bodied peers.

It might appear intuitive that growth in towns would lead to an increase in asylum admissions, but it is more precise to state that the movement of people to towns led to an overextension of welfare provision and consequently increased the number of families struggling to cope. As would be expected, the quantities of children sent to the asylum from the large towns of Northamptonshire reflect such a situation, with Northampton, Kettering and Wellingborough being responsible for 41 % of Berrywood's child admissions. Migration and the change in employment experiences impacted on the traditional care that mentally disabled children would have received in the rural home earlier in the century. As a consequence economic depression was more acutely felt in towns. In this instance the asylum can be viewed as a tool that relieved overburdened families in times of extreme need.

Children were, therefore, not deposited in asylums because they were unproductive, but because their families had limited access to assistance. The workhouses of these towns were flooded with families struggling to cope. The Revd G. Harrison summed up the situation, in 1883, when he lamented that 'it was utterly impossible for a man with a family of small children to provide for their wants, and pay the heavy rates and taxes that were demanded'.[40] It can be safely assumed, considering the importance of a child's contribution to the household economy of the poor, that these demands must have increased exponentially if one or more of their children suffered from a mental illness or disability.[41]

The links between families in crisis and asylum admissions are important, but the impact of urbanisation in Northamptonshire should not be overestimated. It only affected certain parts of the county and the rural character of Northamptonshire persisted well in to the twentieth century.[42] There was, however, a relationship between population movement, the asylum, and child patients. The asylums serving established urban cities received fewer children than those in rural areas or with immature industry. It can be argued, therefore, that an asylum was utilised at specific times in the evolution of its surrounding environment, before the development and expansion of other specific provisions for children that will be explored later. Consequently, the experience of insane children was to some degree shaped by wider social forces and it will be demonstrated in the rest of the chapter how these manifested inside the institution.

Before moving on it is crucial not to overlook the experience of insanity in industrial areas. Lancashire as a county was second only to Middlesex in confining large numbers of the insane. Cox, Marland, and York have shown that Irish migration was a major contributor to the swelling of Lancashire's four pauper lunatic asylums and workhouses, and thus had an impact on policies towards the insane.[43] The LAB was reluctant to send harmless and incurable child cases to the asylum and the insane child was more likely to be confined in a workhouse lunatic ward if they were institutionalised. While Poor Law unions in the Manchester area reluctantly accepted the situation, they were less understanding about paying for the costs of caring for insane children. The Leigh Union complained to the LAB in 1894 about the presence of insane children in their workhouse and the lack of extra institutional space to confine them.[44] Their attitude towards children was shared by other unions in Lancashire, such as Ulverston, West Derby, and Chorlton. Thus highlighting a paradox between our rural and urban asylums that has already been unearthed; with children being pulled into the Northamptonshire Asylum for financial reasons and the Prestwich Asylum resisting the admission of children, despite external pressure from the local Poor Law Unions.

Urbanisation meant that established towns and cities, such as Birmingham and Manchester, had developed a range of responses to poverty and sickness beyond overcrowded workhouses and asylums. For example, there were children's hospitals in all three of the urban centres that feature here. These give physical embodiment to specific medical responses aimed at the young. Charities to deal with a host of disadvantaged populations also emerged during the period. In London there were numerous organisations such as the Church of England Waifs and Strays Society and Barnados to name two of the largest, and in Manchester there was the Manchester and Salford Boys' and Girls' Refuge and religious attempts at 'rescue' promoted by the Roman Catholic Diocese. These avenues of relief reveal a familiarity with poverty on a large scale that led to a growth in mechanisms to deal with the disadvantaged and marginalised, of which insane children were included. Now we turn attention to the children themselves and explore how differences between the urban and rural were contributory factors in their varying experiences.

Profiling Asylum Children

It has been demonstrated that child populations were not large and that there were notable variations in the number of children admitted to each institution. An important, and to some degree surprising observation, is that the industrial cities of Birmingham and Manchester admitted fewer children than the rural asylums of Northampton and Three Counties. Prominent nineteenth-century alienists such as John C. Bucknill, D.H. Tuke, and W.A.F. Browne had posited that rural and agricultural populations were 'to a great degree exempt from insanity'.[45] In their opinions, the amount of time spent active and outdoors combined with a small, yet reliable, income meant that the agricultural classes were not exposed to the 'excitements' that affected more mobile or affluent social classes. Modern scholars have adopted a similar approach and implied that the increased confinement of the insane was a by-product of a capitalist society, with confinement being most frequent in industrial and urban centres where ties of kinship and paternalism had broken down.[46] From the examination of the wider socio-economic context of asylums these arguments have proven inaccurate, at least for the admission of children. In Fig. 3.3 the years when children were admitted to each of the five institutions has been plotted. It reveals a pattern of consistent admission

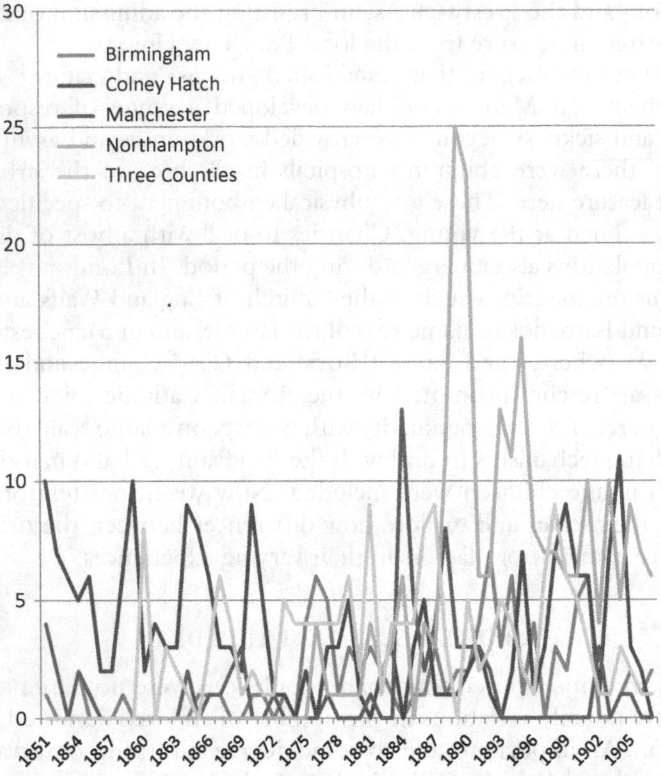

Fig. 3.3 Admissions to each asylum between 1845 and 1907. *Source*: BCL, Male Patient Casebooks, MS344/12/2 & 2a, MS344/12/5, MS344/12/7-9, MS344/12/11-14, MS344/12/20-22, MS344/12/27; BCL, Female Patient Casebooks, MS344/12/41-47, MS344/12/49-51, MS344/12/53 & 54, MS344/12/56 & 57, MS344/12/60-63; BCL, Patient Index, MS344/11/1 & 2; LMA, Colney Hatch Male Patient Casebooks, H12/CH/B/13/001-61; LMA, Colney Hatch Female Patient Casebooks, H12/CH/B/11/001-085; NRO, Male Patient Casebooks, NCLA/6/2/2/1-12; NRO Female Patient Casebooks, NCLA/6/2/1/1-13; GMCRO, Male Patient Casebooks, ADMM/2/1-16; GMCRO, ADMF/2/1-21; LRO, Male Patient Casebooks, QAM/6/6/1-34; LRO, Female Patient Casebooks, QAM/6/6/1-34; BLAS, Male Patient Casebooks, LF31/1-12; BLAS, Female Patient Casebooks, LF29/1-12

throughout the period and demonstrates that children were considered suitable patients to all of the asylums across the chronological period.

It can also be noted that children were admitted regularly to asylums. The Northamptonshire Asylum witnessed an influx related to the opening of its Children's Block which accounts for the large spike in the mid 1880s, but the others display a picture of steady admissions. We must, however, look in more depth to build more detailed profiles of the children that populated asylums. In the Devon County Asylum it was argued that the children confined tended to be male and nearing adolescence, while younger children rarely found their way to the institution.[47] To be able to offer a comparison, the ages of children that entered each institution are plotted in Fig. 3.4.

There evidently were similarities with Devon. The urban asylums of Colney Hatch and Prestwich confined mainly older and what might be described as more boisterous children; such as William Langley, admitted to Colney Hatch, aged twelve, in 1858 because he threatened to stab and kill his mother.[48] But Fig. 3.4 also reveals a high percentage of those aged between eleven and thirteen in all institutions, although they were not as dominant in the asylums at Birmingham, Northamptonshire and Three Counties. In this regard, the contrast with the findings of the Devon institution is striking. At Birmingham the average age at admission was nine, Northampton was just under nine, and Three Counties was slightly over nine. This compares with just below eleven at Colney Hatch, nearly eleven and a half at Manchester, and ten at the Devon County Asylum.[49] The asylum at Birmingham stands out somewhat in the examination of child ages at admission. It was not as heavily dominated by older children like the asylums at Colney Hatch and Prestwich, but its age distribution was not as smooth as those evident at Northamptonshire or Three Counties. Across all of the asylums it is clearly inaccurate to assume that children approaching adolescence were the most likely admissions; rather it is evident that the asylum was used to confine children across the age range with the age of seven appearing to be a point when admissions accelerated. This raises an issue that is worth exploring. In the Catholic Church the age of reason is commonly thought to begin at around this age and symbolically children can begin to take Eucharist. Even though this is not a steadfast ecclesiastic rule, a similar age is used in the Protestant Church for children to take Communion. Therefore an increase in admissions from the age of seven is not just a coincidence or an arbitrary age when parents or doctors believed it was time for a child to be confined, but instead a reaction to an

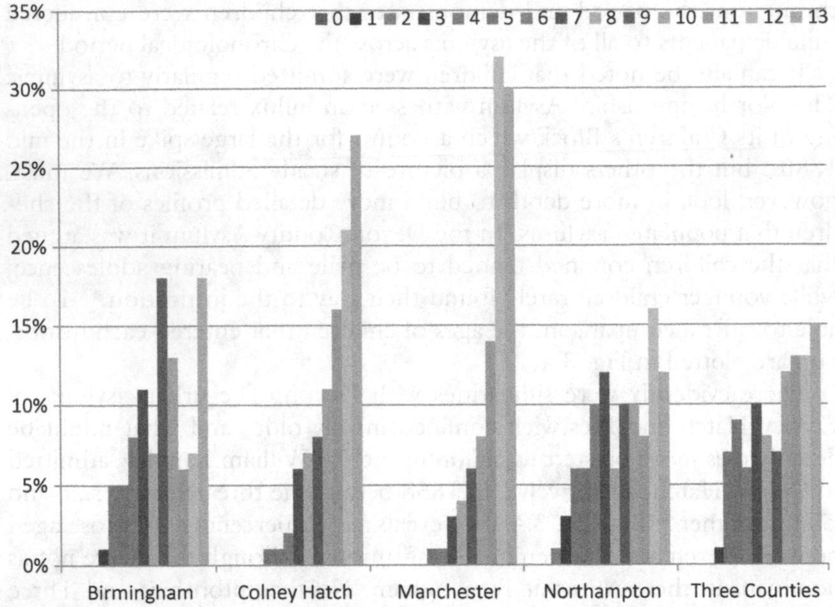

Fig. 3.4 Ages at admission by institution. *Source*: BCL, Male Patient Casebooks, MS344/12/2 & 2a, MS344/12/5, MS344/12/7-9, MS344/12/11-14, MS344/12/20-22, MS344/12/27; BCL, Female Patient Casebooks, MS344/12/41-47, MS344/12/49-51, MS344/12/53 & 54, MS344/12/56 & 57, MS344/12/60-63; BCL, Patient Index, MS344/11/1 & 2; LMA, Colney Hatch Male Patient Casebooks, H12/CH/B/13/001-61; LMA, Colney Hatch Female Patient Casebooks, H12/CH/B/11/001-085; NRO, Male Patient Casebooks, NCLA/6/2/2/1-12; NRO Female Patient Casebooks, NCLA/6/2/1/1-13; GMCRO, Male Patient Casebooks, ADMM/2/1-16; GMCRO, ADMF/2/1-21; LRO, Male Patient Casebooks, QAM/6/6/1-34; LRO, Female Patient Casebooks, QAM/6/6/1-34; BLAS, Male Patient Casebooks, LF31/1-12; BLAS, Female Patient Casebooks, LF29/1-12

individual's lack of 'reason' and confirmation that they would be unable to participate in religious communities in the expected manner. Also, the age of seven was an important watershed in a medical context. Children were never ubiquitous in the voluntary hospitals of the nineteenth century but those younger than this age were excluded from treatment inside them. The age of seven may have also represented an acceptable professional demarcation for medical men to treat and institutionalise individuals.

By further exploring the profiles of children confined inside asylums it becomes evident that the issue of gender encompassed equal complexity as that of age. It has already been demonstrated that male outnumbered female admissions. Girls were most likely fewer in number because they were more useful domestically than males; those that suffered from chronic and harmless conditions could still partake in household chores and offer some limited childcare options.[50] Consequently, it might be expected that girls were admitted to asylums either at an early age, when they were the eldest child in the family and there was limited childcare provision for them, or when they were older and it was apparent they were unable to fend for themselves following the loss of a parent or a shift in the family dynamic.[51] Either way it is clear that there is a wider narrative of family breakdown, either through illness, unemployment or loss, as a push factor in asylum admissions.

By continuing to focus on female admissions we can see that differences between rural and urban asylums are evident (Fig. 3.5). Girls were most likely to be admitted to urban asylums when they were aged between ten and thirteen, while at the rural Three Counties Asylum the average age at admission was also thirteen, but in Northamptonshire the age of seven was most common. At both rural institutions it can be observed that the age distribution was again smoother than urban asylums.

The experience was similar for boys (Fig. 3.6). The urban institutions of Colney Hatch and Prestwich admitted a high percentage of older male patients, much like in Devon. Although, the modal age for a male child confined at Birmingham was nine, this compares with a peak of twelve in Northampton, and eleven at Three Counties. However, the two rural institutions again display a smoother age distribution than those presented for urban institutions. With the children admitted to these asylums it would be too simplistic to suggest that the institution merely regulated the behaviour of adolescent males. Also there was not a vast difference in experience between the sexes at admission. Therefore variations need to be framed typologically or regionally, rather than by gender or age.

We know that the majority of children in the patient sample were diagnosed with the mental disabilities of idiocy or imbecility. Looking at how asylums explained the causes of insanity aids judgments about the position that children and their illnesses held inside them. This approach reveals further typological divergences between rural and urban institutions. In the Birmingham, Colney Hatch, and Prestwich Asylums the perceived cause of a child's mental disability was recorded in only 23 %, 39 %, and

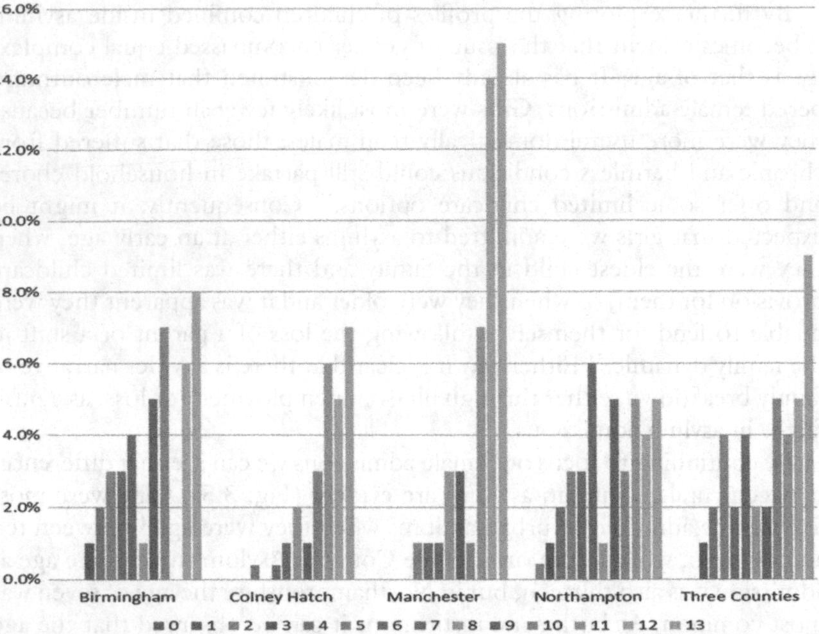

Fig. 3.5 Female ages at admission by institution. *Source*: BCL, Male Patient Casebooks, MS344/12/2 & 2a, MS344/12/5, MS344/12/7-9, MS344/12/11-14, MS344/12/20-22, MS344/12/27; BCL, Female Patient Casebooks, MS344/12/41-47, MS344/12/49-51, MS344/12/53 & 54, MS344/12/56 & 57, MS344/12/60-63; BCL, Patient Index, MS344/11/1 & 2; LMA, Colney Hatch Male Patient Casebooks, H12/CH/B/13/001-61; LMA, Colney Hatch Female Patient Casebooks, H12/CH/B/11/001-085; NRO, Male Patient Casebooks, NCLA/6/2/2/1-12; NRO Female Patient Casebooks, NCLA/6/2/1/1-13; GMCRO, Male Patient Casebooks, ADMM/2/1-16; GMRCO, ADMF/2/1-21; LRO, Male Patient Casebooks, QAM/6/6/1-34; LRO, Female Patient Casebooks, QAM/6/6/1-34; BLAS, Male Patient Casebooks, LF31/1-12; BLAS, Female Patient Casebooks, LF29/1-12

29 % of cases respectively. By contrast the asylum in Northamptonshire recorded causative explanations in 50 % of cases and Three Counties 42 %. The manageable number of children makes it possible to glean such detailed information from the processes of admission used at each asylum. The institutional breakdown for each causative category is presented in Table 3.1. Here we can observe that 'no cause recorded' was the largest

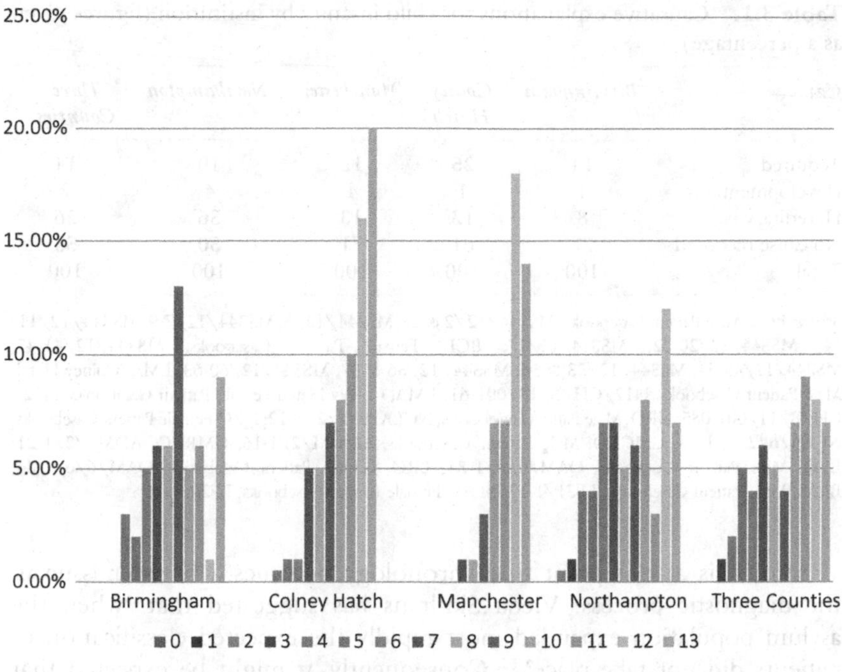

Fig. 3.6 Male ages at admission by institution. *Source*: BCL, Male Patient Casebooks, MS344/12/2 & 2a, MS344/12/5, MS344/12/7-9, MS344/12/11-14, MS344/12/20-22, MS344/12/27; BCL, Female Patient Casebooks, MS344/12/41-47, MS344/12/49-51, MS344/12/53 & 54, MS344/12/56 & 57, MS344/12/60-63; BCL, Patient Index, MS344/11/1 & 2; LMA, Colney Hatch Male Patient Casebooks, H12/CH/B/13/001-61; LMA, Colney Hatch Female Patient Casebooks, H12/CH/B/11/001-085; NRO, Male Patient Casebooks, NCLA/6/2/2/1-12; NRO Female Patient Casebooks, NCLA/6/2/1/1-13; GMCRO, Male Patient Casebooks, ADMM/2/1-16; GMRCO, ADMF/2/1-21; LRO, Male Patient Casebooks, QAM/6/6/1-34; LRO, Female Patient Casebooks, QAM/6/6/1-34; BLAS, Male Patient Casebooks, LF31/1-12; BLAS, Female Patient Casebooks, LF29/1-12

category, suggesting that asylums either found it difficult to assign a cause or doctors were indifferent to the aetiological roots of child mental disability. Rural asylums, with their slower patient turnover, seem to have put more time into seeking explanations and it might be assumed that they had a better understanding of child conditions than their urban contemporaries.

Table 3.1. Causative explanations for child insanity by institution (figures given as a percentage)

Cause	*Birmingham*	*Colney Hatch*	*Manchester*	*Northampton*	*Three Counties*
Acquired	14	25	12	10	14
Developmental	1	1	4	4	2
Hereditary	8	13	13	36	26
No cause recorded	77	61	71	50	58
Total	100	100	100	100	100

Source: BCL, Male Patient Casebooks, MS344/12/2 & 2a, MS344/12/5, MS344/12/7-9, MS344/12/11-14, MS344/12/20-22, MS344/12/27; BCL, Female Patient Casebooks, MS344/12/41-47, MS344/12/49-51, MS344/12/53 & 54, MS344/12/56 & 57, MS344/12/60-63; LMA, Colney Hatch Male Patient Casebooks, H12/CH/B/13/001-61; LMA, Colney Hatch Female Patient Casebooks, H12/CH/B/11/001-085; NRO, Male Patient Casebooks, NCLA/6/2/2/1-12; NRO Female Patient Casebooks, NCLA/6/2/1/1-13; GMCRO, Male Patient Casebooks, ADMM/2/1-16; GMRCO, ADMF/2/1-21; LRO, Male Patient Casebooks, QAM/6/6/1-34; LRO, Female Patient Casebooks, QAM/6/6/1-34; BLAS, Male Patient Casebooks, LF31/1-12; BLAS, Female Patient Casebooks, LF29/1-12

Also, it is at this point that chronology becomes a broader issue in the diagnostic process. Vieda Skultans has suggested that 'when the asylum population expanded most rapidly the expected classification of patients did not take place'.[52] Consequently, it might be expected that the majority of causes would be recorded at the beginning of an asylum's life before the fatigue of overcrowding had dampened the curative ambitions of the institution. Plotting the years when causative explanations were recorded demonstrates that such a suggestion is problematic. While it is indisputable that asylums became overcrowded, the 1862 Lunacy Acts Amendment Act sought to relieve the pressure on asylums by permitting workhouses to house some of the pauper insane that were diagnosed as chronic and harmless. It is confirmed by Fig. 3.7 that causative explanations for child mental disability occurred throughout the period and those with hereditary causes were in fact recorded more regularly as the period progressed. The increase can again be explained by the growing influence of eugenicists, especially considering the impact and influence of psychiatrists such as Henry Maudsley who were supportive of policies such as selective breeding. In relation to adult asylum patients it is unclear if a similar pattern of hereditary causes would develop as they were less likely to be admitted suffering from the harmless and incurable conditions presented by children.

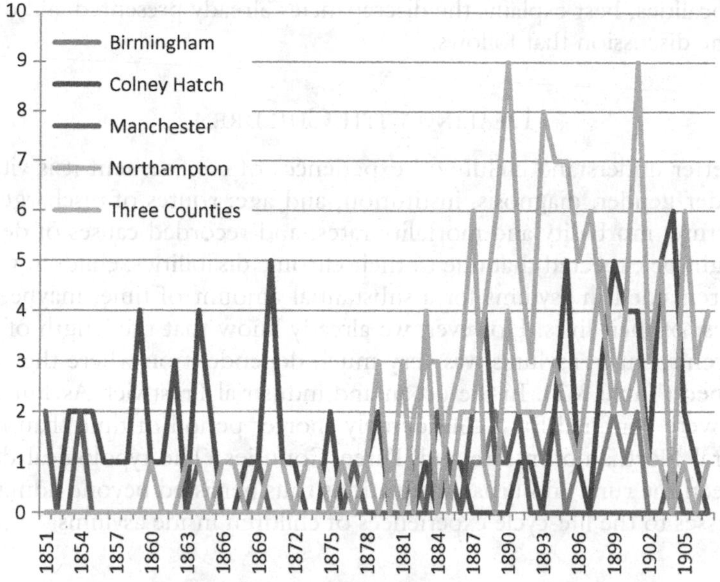

Fig. 3.7 The occurrence of causative explanations for child patients by asylum. *Source*: BCL, Male Patient Casebooks, MS344/12/2 & 2a, MS344/12/5, MS344/12/7-9, MS344/12/11-14, MS344/12/20-22, MS344/12/27; BCL, Female Patient Casebooks, MS344/12/41-47, MS344/12/49-51, MS344/12/53 & 54, MS344/12/56 & 57, MS344/12/60-63; LMA, Colney Hatch Male Patient Casebooks, H12/CH/B/13/001-61; LMA, Colney Hatch Female Patient Casebooks, H12/CH/B/11/001-085; NRO, Male Patient Casebooks, NCLA/6/2/2/1-12; NRO Female Patient Casebooks, NCLA/6/2/1/1-13; GMCRO, Male Patient Casebooks, ADMM/2/1-16; GMRCO, ADMF/2/1-21; LRO, Male Patient Casebooks, QAM/6/6/1-34; LRO, Female Patient Casebooks, QAM/6/6/1-34; BLAS, Male Patient Casebooks, LF31/1-12; BLAS, Female Patient Casebooks, LF29/1-12

It would be easy to attribute the discrepancies between the urban and rural to random variations in practice due to the small numbers, but that would be to dismiss the subtle differences that occurred between institutions. The best explanation for fluctuations in experience is to conclude that the catchment areas of urban and rural institutions were vital in framing the experiences of each type of institution. Adopting a typological approach, rather than a regional one that seeks differences amongst all of our localities, best explains the discrepancies already presented and develops the discussion that follows.

Dealing with Children

To better understand childhood experiences of confinement it is vital to consider gender, diagnosis, institution, and age; routes of discharge and departure; morbidity and mortality rates; and recorded causes of deaths. It might be expected that due to their chronic disabilities, children would have remained in asylums for a substantial amount of time, maybe even the rest of their lives. However, we already know that the length of time children spent in asylums was very much dependent on where they were confined (Table 3.2). In the urban and industrial Prestwich Asylum children were confined for a considerably shorter period of time than those in rural Northamptonshire and Three Counties. The typological divide between the rural and urban institutions thus persisted beyond admission processes to the life-cycle experiences of children inside asylums.

Table 3.2 Average duration of stay for child patients by institution. (Length of time is represented by a decimal figure e.g. 7.6 is equivalent to 7 years and 6 months)

	Birmingham	*Colney Hatch*	*Manchester*	*Northampton*	*Three Counties*
Sample avg	2.10	4.6	.10	6.5	7.6
Female/male avgs	2.6/3.3	4.11/4.1	1/0.8	6.8/6.2	7.9/7.3
Causative avg	1.3	2.8	0.10	5.11	4.1
Causative F/M	1/1.6	1.8/3.6	1.2/0.6	6.5/5.4	5/3.2

Note: The table is broken down into the collective sample average, collective sample gender averages and then by an average duration of stay for those with a causative explanation for their condition. The final row shows the causative average subdivided further by gender.

Source: BCL, Male Patient Casebooks, MS344/12/2 & 2a, MS344/12/5, MS344/12/7-9, MS344/12/11-14, MS344/12/20-22, MS344/12/27; BCL, Female Patient Casebooks, MS344/12/41-47, MS344/12/49-51, MS344/12/53 & 54, MS344/12/56 & 57, MS344/12/60-63; LMA, Colney Hatch Male Patient Casebooks, H12/CH/B/13/001-61; LMA, Colney Hatch Female Patient Casebooks, H12/CH/B/11/001-085; NRO, Male Patient Casebooks, NCLA/6/2/2/1-12; NRO Female Patient Casebooks, NCLA/6/2/1/1-13; GMCRO, Male Patient Casebooks, ADMM/2/1-16; GMRCO, ADMF/2/1-21; LRO, Male Patient Casebooks, QAM/6/6/1-34; LRO, Female Patient Casebooks, QAM/6/6/1-34; BLAS, Male Patient Casebooks, LF31/1-12; BLAS, Female Patient Casebooks, LF29/1-12

Further expanding earlier discussions of age, Fig. 3.8 demonstrates that those aged between seven and nine at admission were confined for the longest periods of time. This reinforces the notion that asylums confined children and not just proto-adults. By way of example, in 1868 John Prutton was admitted to the Three Counties Asylum, aged eight, diagnosed as a congenital imbecile and described as thin, feeble, and mischievous.[53] He remained in the asylum until his death thirty-nine years later. In contrast, Robert Brocklehurst was admitted to the Prestwich asylum in 1866, aged twelve. He was diagnosed as an idiot and described as restless, mischievous, and destructive, however he was discharged after just three months.[54] Whilst these two children had similar diagnoses they experienced the different networks of care available in urban and rural areas, thus personifying the complexity that existed in the management of mentally disabled children. The length of time that children spent in institutions is, however, only one half of the picture. Prutton and Brocklehurst experienced two very different methods of exiting the institution; by exploring departures it is possible to expand our understanding of how asylums operated with regards to this specific patient population. There were numerous routes out of the asylum for children; they could recover, parents or friends could request their removal, they could be discharged as not improved, transferred to another institution, or die. Differences again occurred between rural and urban asylums (Fig. 3.9). Those confined in the rural institutions of Northampton and Three Counties not only spent much longer in the institution but were also more likely to die there, with over 60 % of children dying. In contrast the asylum at Manchester most commonly transferred children to other institutions, a method adopted in all asylums but never on the same scale. The varied functions of asylums are important and the role of the institution as a carousel moving children around the nineteenth-century welfare system is an issue that requires further attention.

One might argue that the deaths of children in the asylum were nothing more than reflections of wider regional trends in mortality and thus are not exceptional. If this was the case, it would be expected that more deaths would have occurred in one institution over another because of these regional factors. If we consider infant mortality rates, the closest age indicator to our child patient's experience, it is possible to make some tentative judgments (Table 3.3). In the counties that were home to our urban institutions infant mortality rates amongst the wider population were considerably higher than those of our rural asylums. Yet there were more child

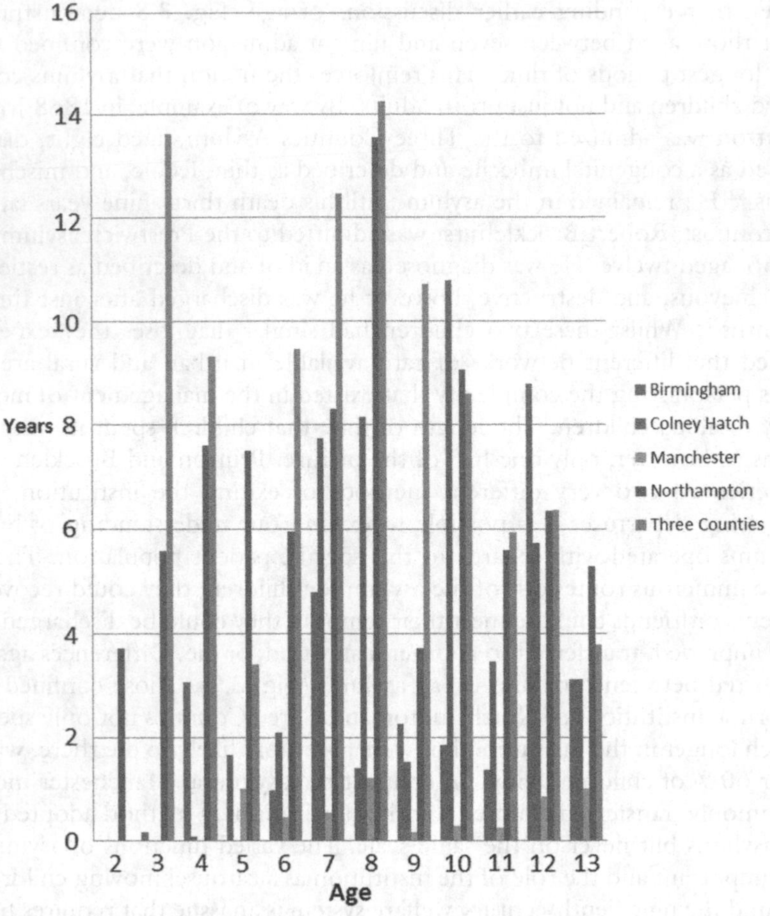

Fig. 3.8 Average duration of stay by institution and age. *Source*: BCL, Male Patient Casebooks, MS344/12/2 & 2a, MS344/12/5, MS344/12/7-9, MS344/12/11-14, MS344/12/20-22, MS344/12/27; BCL, Female Patient Casebooks, MS344/12/41-47, MS344/12/49-51, MS344/12/53 & 54, MS344/12/56 & 57, MS344/12/60-63; BCL, Patient Index, MS344/11/1 & 2; LMA, Colney Hatch Male Patient Casebooks, H12/CH/B/13/001-61; LMA, Colney Hatch Female Patient Casebooks, H12/CH/B/11/001-085; NRO, Male Patient Casebooks, NCLA/6/2/2/1-12; NRO Female Patient Casebooks, NCLA/6/2/1/1-13; GMCRO, Male Patient Casebooks, ADMM/2/1-16; GMCRO, ADMF/2/1-21; LRO, Male Patient Casebooks, QAM/6/6/1-34; LRO, Female Patient Casebooks, QAM/6/6/1-34; BLAS, Male Patient Casebooks, LF31/1-12; BLAS, Female Patient Casebooks, LF29/1-12

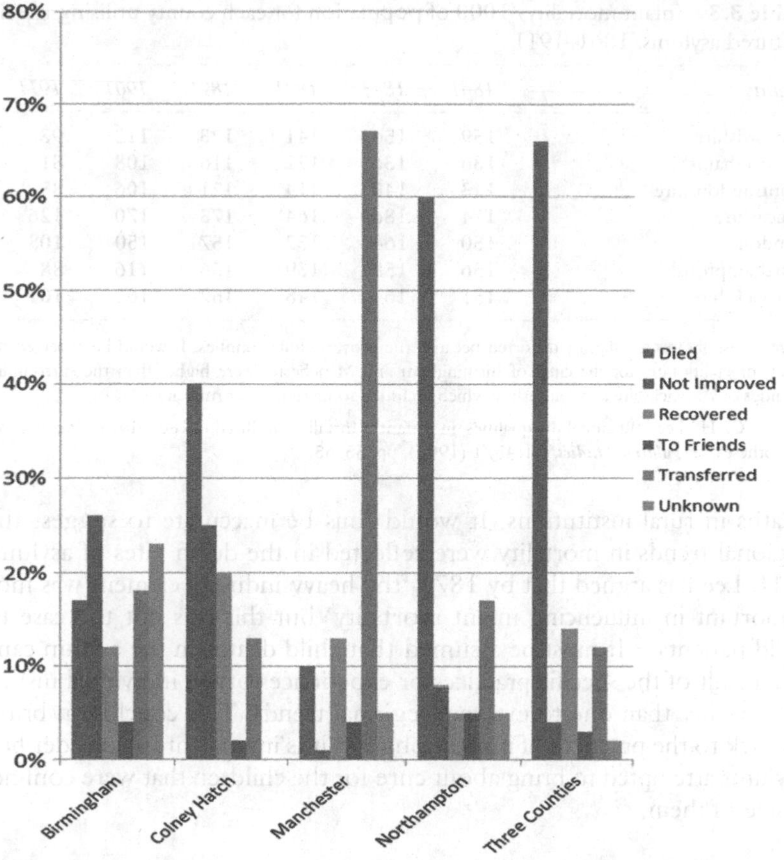

Fig. 3.9 Departures of child patients by institution. *Source*: BCL, Male Patient Casebooks, MS344/12/2 & 2a, MS344/12/5, MS344/12/7-9, MS344/12/11-14, MS344/12/20-22, MS344/12/27; BCL, Female Patient Casebooks, MS344/12/41-47, MS344/12/49-51, MS344/12/53 & 54, MS344/12/56 & 57, MS344/12/60-63; BCL, Patient Index, MS344/11/1 & 2; LMA, Colney Hatch Male Patient Casebooks, H12/CH/B/13/001-61; LMA, Colney Hatch Female Patient Casebooks, H12/CH/B/11/001-085; NRO, Male Patient Casebooks, NCLA/6/2/2/1-12; NRO Female Patient Casebooks, NCLA/6/2/1/1-13; GMCRO, Male Patient Casebooks, ADMM/2/1-16; GMRCO, ADMF/2/1-21; LRO, Male Patient Casebooks, QAM/6/6/1-34; LRO, Female Patient Casebooks, QAM/6/6/1-34; BLAS, Male Patient Casebooks, LF31/1-12; BLAS, Female Patient Casebooks, LF29/1-12

Table 3.3 Infant mortality/1000 of population for each county utilising the five featured asylums, 1861–1911

County	*1861*	*1871*	*1881*	*1891*	*1901*	*1911*
Bedfordshire	159	156	141	123	112	93
Buckinghamshire	136	136	122	116	108	81
Huntingdonshire	143	140	114	121	106	85
Lancashire	174	186	164	173	170	126
London	150	164	152	157	150	108
Northamptonshire	156	158	139	136	116	88
Warwickshire	151	164	148	157	161	101

Note: These figures are slightly distorted because they cover whole counties. It would be expected that infant mortality rates for the cities of Birmingham and Manchester were higher than the surrounding counties of Warwickshire and Lancashire which included some significant rural areas.

Source: C. H. Lee, 'Regional Inequalities in Infant Mortality in Britain, 1861–1971: Patterns and Hypotheses,' *Population Studies*, vol. 45/1 (1991), pp. 55–65.

deaths in rural institutions. It would thus be inaccurate to suggest that regional trends in mortality were reflected in the death rates of asylums. C.H. Lee has argued that by 1871 'the heavy-industry element was most important in influencing infant mortality' but this was not the case for child patients.[55] It must be assumed that child deaths in the asylum came as a result of the specific practices or experiences of the individual institution, rather than due to external regional trends. This conclusion brings us back to the practices of institutions and it is important to consider how asylums attempted to bring about cure for the children that were confined inside of them.

Treatment

Due to the nature of asylum record keeping and the limited psychiatric understanding of child mental health issues it is difficult to gauge the precise type of treatments that children received. Patient casebooks have recorded the medical history of the patient, but these were often detailed notes of physical ailments rather than mental afflictions. Medical treatment tended to be reactive rather than proactive and attention to cleanliness, behaviour, diet, and physical well-being featured most often in the casenotes. Such an approach is not surprising and mirrors the prevalent belief of asylum physicians that good physical health would lead to improved mental well-being. With no reference to age limits or suitable ages for admission, it could simply be argued that the experience of child patients in terms of treatment was similar to that of adults. This, however, is a dangerous assumption to make. In the wider historiography of childhood illness Hannah Newton has observed that as early as the seventeenth century doctors were familiar with treating children and in fact tailored remedies to meet their needs. She has argued that physicians had a distinct idea of the diseases that afflicted the young rather than adults, amongst which epilepsy was included.[56] The argument here has developed along similar lines and it is apparent that there were specific disabilities that children were admitted to asylums with.

Recovery for child patients was unlikely (Fig. 3.9), but improvement in their conditions was thought to be brought about in the asylum through the progressive and humanitarian ideal of moral treatment. The effectiveness of this approach is hard to measure, as asylum populations expanded and became more difficult to manage, key elements of the approach appear to have been overlooked. Anne Borsay has argued that even at the Quaker run York Retreat, a relatively small institution compared to the county pauper facilities, the increase in the numbers of insane meant that by 1870 moral treatment was ineffective and chemical concoctions were increasingly common.[57] Amongst child patients the low recovery rates are indicative of the chronic and incurable disabilities that children were diagnosed with, consequently the impact of moral methods to treat them is somewhat moot. It could be argued in this instance that Scull's view of asylums being used to detain the unproductive and burdensome might hold some weight. It will be demonstrated, however, that children confined in these asylums could be productive and a different measure of 'improvement' needs to be deployed in this instance.

The employment of patients in the asylum was a key feature of moral therapy. Its purpose was to reflect a routine of life comparable to that outside of the institution and to instil notions of contribution and self-worth within the pauper population. By getting patients into the habit of working it was hoped that they would continue such behaviour following their reintroduction into society. This would of course come with the added benefits of easing the financial burden on Poor Law authorities, and the creation of a more productive society.[58] Such utopian expectations were of course difficult to achieve and the fruits of patient labour often aided the institution rather than bringing about the therapeutic goals of moral treatment.[59] The five asylums reveal a mixed approach to work for children. The Northamptonshire and Three Counties Asylums recorded the employment of some children inside the institutions. Boys were often occupied in trades such as carpentry, tailoring or farming, while girls were engaged in sewing, cleaning, and laundry work. For example, at Berrywood Arthur Hillam was employed on the farm, Jane Ball worked in a laundry, and Thomas Thomas was employed in the tailor's shop, although his progress was described as 'infinitesimal'.[60] At Three Counties Asylum, Elizabeth Mead regularly completed needlework, Mary Ann Pilgrim was 'employed about the ward', and Sidney Woodland worked 'at times at tailoring, but rather lazy at it'.[61] While the productivity of children might have been questionable, these efforts, alongside those of adult patients, went a long way to making the asylum a self-sustaining institution. Asylums were not merely receptacles for those unable to function in a capitalist society. The individuals confined inside of them were regularly engaged in a range of tasks and jobs that reduced the daily running expenses of the asylum, a necessity given the low numbers of non-patient staff. Experiences with work for children were not, however, recorded in the urban asylums, but the durations of stay there were considerably shorter. Consequently, it is difficult to build a picture of daily life for children confined inside of them.

The employment of children, of course, has implications for more general ideas about the nature of childhood in the nineteenth century. During the period child labour was considered to be exploitative and ran in direct opposition to the developing romantic ideal of childhood as a time of sheltered innocence. Legislative efforts, such as the Factory Acts (1833–1878) and Elementary Education Acts (1870–1902), were introduced to safeguard exploited youngsters but children with mental impairments were exempt from protective measures because employment was deemed therapeutic, and not dangerous. Child labour, conducted inside asylums, was a clear contradiction of social ideals, but was legitimised by the perceived inability of the mentally impaired to benefit from formal education and by extension a 'normal' childhood. Instead these youngsters received an inappropriate labouring education designed to prepare them for life in a work force that they would most likely never be a part of. There were, however, rare occurrences when county asylums did seek to invest in and educate the mentally disabled. At the Warwick Asylum, Dr Henry Parsey took a special interest in education and built a specialised idiot asylum but this was very much the exception rather than the rule and its success was limited.[62]

Medicinal methods of treating the mental afflictions of children were limited. As well as children being more likely to die in rural institutions than urban, they were also more likely to succumb to diseases associated with poverty such as consumption, phthisis, and tuberculosis, rather than mental ailments, giving the sense of the asylum as hospice in these areas (Tables 3.4 and 3.5). The most common explanations for the death of children in asylums were epilepsy and lung diseases, neither of which were illnesses supposed to be confined in these institutions. It is also evident that the records of urban asylums are blighted by a failure to regularly record the causes that led to death. This is a possible symptom of children being considered inferior patients and receiving less medical attention than adults.

When patients received medicinal treatment it was designed to relieve symptoms rather than bring about recovery. For instance, potassium bromide was regularly used as a sedative to aid sleep and to control the symptoms of epilepsy. Evidence of children receiving medicine appears frequently in the records, but details of how they were deployed might appear vague to the modern observer. At the Three Counties Asylum it was noted in 1884 that William Clarvis 'now keeps well at night, without the aid of drugs';[63] suggesting that previously he had been reliant on medication to sleep. Also Samuel Parish was regularly administered seven and a half grams of chloral hydrate for epileptic fits and Kate Chapman took 'thyroid tablets'.[64] The varied application of medicinal relief suggests that asylums were used to care for an array of medical conditions, including those slowly declining from physical illnesses.

Table 3.4 Causes of death for child patients (mental health explanations)

Cause of death	*Birmingham*	*Colney Hatch*	*Manchester*	*Northampton*	*Three Counties*	*Total*
Brain disease	1	2	0	17	5	25
Epilepsy	0	9	3	28	24	64
Idiocy	0	2	0	2	0	4
General paralysis	1	2	0	2	1	6
Hydrocephalous	0	1	0	1	0	2
Total	2	16	3	50	30	101

Source: BCL, Male Patient Casebooks, MS344/12/2 & 2a, MS344/12/5, MS344/12/7-9, MS344/12/11-14, MS344/12/20-22, MS344/12/27; BCL, Female Patient Casebooks, MS344/12/41-47, MS344/12/49-51, MS344/12/53 & 54, MS344/12/56 & 57, MS344/12/60-63; BCL, Patient Index, MS344/11/1 & 2; LMA, Colney Hatch Male Patient Casebooks, H12/CH/B/13/001-61; LMA, Colney Hatch Female Patient Casebooks, H12/CH/B/11/001-085; NRO, Male Patient Casebooks, NCLA/6/2/2/1-12; NRO Female Patient Casebooks, NCLA/6/2/1/1-13; GMCRO, Male Patient Casebooks, ADMM/2/1-16; GMCRO, ADMF/2/1-21; LRO, Male Patient Casebooks, QAM/6/6/1-34; LRO, Female Patient Casebooks, QAM/6/6/1-34; BLAS, Male Patient Casebooks, LF31/1-12; BLAS, Female Patient Casebooks, LF29/1-12

Table 3.5 Causes of death for child patients (physical explanations)

Cause of death	*Birmingham*	*Colney Hatch*	*Manchester*	*Northampton*	*Three Counties*	*Total*
Lung diseases	3	9	2	50	27	91
Diarrhoea	0	1	0	0	0	1
Exhaustion	0	3	0	1	1	5
Pneumonia	0	3	0	9	7	19
Erysipelas	0	0	0	1	0	1
Syphilis	0	0	0	1	0	1
Scarlet fever	0	0	0	1	0	1
Kidney disease	0	0	0	1	3	4
Malnutrition	0	0	0	1	3	4
Accidental	0	1	0	1	1	3
Unknown	10	52	1	14	17	94
Total	13	69	3	80	59	224

Note: For the purposes of keeping the table a manageable size some of the fields have been condensed. The lung diseases category contains a range of degenerative conditions such as phthisis, consumption, and tuberculosis. Often these terms were synonymous and so do not distort the analysis. Similarly brain diseases such as cerebral palsy, meningitis and tumours have been listed as a single category to encompass a range of cerebral conditions that were often recorded in small numbers.

Source: BCL, Male Patient Casebooks, MS344/12/2 & 2a, MS344/12/5, MS344/12/7-9, MS344/12/11-14, MS344/12/20-22, MS344/12/27; BCL, Female Patient Casebooks, MS344/12/41-47, MS344/12/49-51, MS344/12/53 & 54, MS344/12/56 & 57, MS344/12/60-63; BCL, Patient Index, MS344/11/1 & 2; LMA, Colney Hatch Male Patient Casebooks, H12/CH/B/13/001-61; LMA, Colney Hatch Female Patient Casebooks, H12/CH/B/11/001-085; NRO, Male Patient Casebooks, NCLA/6/2/2/1-12; NRO Female Patient Casebooks, NCLA/6/2/1/1-13; GMCRO, Male Patient Casebooks, ADMM/2/1-16; GMCRO, ADMF/2/1-21; LRO, Male Patient Casebooks, QAM/6/6/1-34; LRO, Female Patient Casebooks, QAM/6/6/1-34; BLAS, Male Patient Casebooks, LF31/1-12; BLAS, Female Patient Casebooks, LF29/1-12

Colney Hatch took in seven children who died within three months of entering the institution, all from non-mental health related diseases. At Birmingham Thomas Skirrow was admitted, aged eleven, in 1892. He was diagnosed as an imbecile but had died within five months from phthisis. His illness must have been evident long before he found his way to the asylum and his stay was dominated by attempts to relieve his physical ailments. Skirrow was put to bed and his temperature regularly checked, there were efforts to make him comfortable but attempts at bringing about recovery were impossible.[65] In 1886, Caroline Clements was admitted to the Northamptonshire Asylum, with the prognosis of 'death from phthisis within three years', she duly died from the condition eighteen months later.[66] At Three Counties, George Clark was sent to the asylum in 1876 diagnosed as an epileptic 'suffering from phthisis'. He died in the institution ten years later, the cause of death recorded as general tuberculosis.[67] From these examples it is evident that the asylum was utilised as both a short and long-term option for the treatment of non-mental health conditions.

A broad range of mental and physical illness evidently coalesced inside asylums. Those responsible for the care of patients were faced with finite resources and training to deal with them. Therefore responses to child patients were limited. Children suffering from a mental disability or physical illness were allowed access to specialist attention and the nursing that they required, but beyond that there was very little that could be offered. Asylums may have been established as institutions of cure for child patients, however, and particularly in rural areas, they were accessed as spaces of care and custody.

Conclusion

The sustained and systematic difference in the function of the urban and rural asylums towards insane children raises a number of questions about the network of these institutions during the period. Variation between rural and urban practice is evident at every level of analysis and it is clear that there was no common asylum approach towards child patients. These were embedded in the broader social and economic structures of the areas and extended beyond medical discourses towards the mentally ill. Consequently, we can see that a national asylum system did not exist during the period, but instead there was a network of county institutions linked by legislation and not necessarily through medical practice. Until now the impact of external socio-economic factors on methods for dealing with the insane has not been adequately developed.

It has been demonstrated that there were systematic typological differences in how asylums catered for child patients. While Melling et al. had suggested that children remained outside of pauper asylums, it has been shown that this argument cannot be extrapolated to a national picture.[68] The asylums examined here clearly had different approaches to the management of child insanity. Our industrial and urban institutions pushed insane children away from the asylum and they were subjected to other methods of provisions. The asylums located in rural and developing industrial areas were, however, more receptive to the insane child; with the asylum at Northampton actively seeking out the admission of children for its own financial benefit.

Also, ideas about the types of children found in asylums have been developed. While the literature has argued that the asylum functioned as a place to confine young adolescents, the experience here suggests that this was not the case. County asylums operated for children through the age range, with rural areas displaying a more even distribution across ages , reflecting the more limited alternatives in these areas to treat children. We also observe a mixed function for the asylum. In rural areas it was more likely that they acted as receptacles for those struggling to cope. In contrast, industrial regions did not have high rates of admission, suggesting that child confinement was linked to social development and experience. Furthermore, the impact of wider influences on individual institutions such as the drive to cut costs in Northampton has not been considered by historians. The Berrywood asylum pulled children towards the institution, while Manchester pushed them away, resulting in insane children being cared for in alternative arrangements. The suggestion that increased numbers of the insane were a by-product of industrialisation and urbanisation needs to be explored in a wider institutional context. Questions about the nature of medical provisions for the mentally impaired in the welfare landscape and accessibility are issues that need to be examined in more depth. But now the focus alters slightly to consider the role of the pauper lunatic asylum in a broader landscape of care and how this impacted upon children.

Notes

1. B. Forsythe, J. Melling, and R. Adair, 'The New Poor Law and the County Pauper Lunatic Asylum—The Devon Experience 1834–1884,' *Social History of Medicine*, 9/3 (1996), pp. 335–355; Adair, Melling, and Forsythe, 'Migration, Family Structure and Pauper Lunacy in Victorian England: Admissions to the Devon County Pauper Lunatic Asylum, 1845–1900,' *Continuity and Change*, 12/3 (1997), pp. 373–401; Melling, Adair, and Forsythe, '"A Proper Lunatic for Two Years": Pauper Lunatic Children in Victorian and Edwardian England. Child Admissions to the Devon County Asylum, 1845–1914,' *Journal of Social History*, 31/2 (1997), pp. 371–405; Adair, Forsythe, and Melling, 'A Danger to the Public? Disposing of Pauper Lunatics in Late-Victorian and Edwardian England: Plympton St Mary Union and the Devon County Asylum, 1867–1914,' *Medical History*, 42/1 (1998), pp. 1–25.
2. C. Cox, H. Marland, and S. York, 'Emaciated, Exhausted and Excited: The Bodies and Minds of the Irish in Late Nineteenth-Century Lancashire

Asylums,' *Journal of Social History*, 46/2, pp. 500–524; Cox, Marland, and York, 'Itineraries and Experiences of Insanity: Irish Migration and the Management of Mental Illness in Nineteenth-Century Lancashire,' in Cox and Marland (eds.), *Migration, Health and Ethnicity in the Modern World* (Basingstoke: Palgrave Macmillan, 2013), pp. 36–60.

3. R. Ellis, 'The Asylum, the Poor Law and the Growth of County Asylums in Nineteenth-Century Yorkshire,' *Northern History*, 45/2 (2008), pp. 279–293; Ellis, 'The Asylum, the Poor Law, and a Reassessment of the Four-Shilling Grant: Admissions to the County Asylums of Yorkshire in the Nineteenth Century,' *Social History of Medicine*, 19/1 (2006), pp. 55–71; C. Smith, 'Parsimony, Power, and Prescriptive Legislation: The Politics of Pauper Lunacy in Northamptonshire, 1845–1876,' *Bulletin of the History of Medicine*, 81/2 (2007), pp. 359–385; 'Family, Community and the Victorian Asylum: A Case Study of the Northampton General Lunatic Asylum and its Pauper Lunatics,' *Family and Community History*, 9/2 (2006), pp. 109–124; 'Living with Insanity: Narratives of Poverty, Pauperism and Sickness in Asylum Records 1840–76,' in A. Gestrich, E. Hurren, and S. King (eds.), *Poverty and Sickness in Modern Europe: Narratives of the Sick Poor*, 1780–1938, pp. 117–142; D. Wright, *Mental Disability in Victorian England: The Earlswood Asylum, 1847–1901* (Oxford: Clarendon, 2001); Wright, '"Childlike in His Innocence": Lay Attitudes to "Idiots" and "Imbecilies" in Victorian England,' in A. Digby and D. Wright (eds.), *From Idiocy to Mental Deficiency: Historical Perspectives on People with Learning Disabilities* (London: Routledge, 1996), pp. 118–133; Wright, 'Getting Out of the Asylum: Understanding the Confinement of the Insane in the Nineteenth Century,' *Social History of Medicine*, 10/1 (1997), pp. 137–155; D. Gladstone, 'The Changing Dynamic of Institutional Care: The Western Counties Idiot Asylum, 1864–1914,' in D. Wright and A. Digby (eds.), *From Idiocy to Mental Deficiency*, pp. 134–160.
4. A. Scull, *Museums of Madness: The Social Organisation of Insanity in Nineteenth-Century England* (London: Allen Lane, 1979), p. 16.
5. C. Smith, 'Parsimony, Power and Local Politics'; E. Hurren, *Protesting about Pauperism: Poverty, Politics and Poor Relief in Late-Victorian England, 1870–1900* (Woodbridge: Boydell & Brewer, 2007).
6. Ellis, 'The Asylum, the Poor Law'.
7. NRO, Annual Report of the Northampton County Lunatic Asylum at Berry Wood, near Northampton for the year 1880 (Northampton: Cordex and Sons, 1881), p. 3.
8. E. Hurren, *Dying for Victorian Medicine: English Anatomy and its Trade in the Dead Poor* (London: Palgrave Macmillan, 2011), p. 136.
9. NRO, Annual Report, 1888, p. 2.

10. NRO, Memorandum Prepared by the Medical Superintendent for the Committee of Visitors, NCLA/1/2/2/1/5.
11. NRO, Account Book for Nursing Staff and Servants, NCLA/5/2/2/1.
12. GMCRO, Proceedings of the Lancashire Asylums Board and arrival Reports of County Asylums, A/Pres/Box 647 1894–1912.
13. GMCRO, Proceedings of the Lancashire Asylums Board and arrival Reports of County Asylums, A/Pres/Box 647, 28 February 1895.
14. Ibid.
15. Ibid., 29 August 1895.
16. Ibid., 25 February 1897.
17. N.L. Tranter, *Population Since the Industrial Revolution: The Case of England and Wales* (London: Croom Helm 1973); Eric Lampard, 'The Urbanizing World,' in H.J. Dyos and M. Wolff (eds.), *The Victorian City: Images and Realities*, vol. 1 (London: Routledge & Kegan Paul Ltd, 1973), pp. 3–58; R.J. Morris, 'Urbanization,' in R.J. Morris and R. Rodger (eds.), *The Victorian City: A Reader in British Urban History 1820–1914* (London: Longman, 1993), pp. 43–72; E.A. Wrigley, *Poverty, Progress, and Population* (Cambridge: Cambridge University Press, 2004); J. Stobart and N. Raven, "Introduction: Industrialisation and Urbanisation in a Regional Context,' in J. Stobart and N. Raven (eds.), *Towns, Regions and Industries: Urban and Industrial Change, 1700–1840* (Manchester: Manchester University Press, 2005).
18. Wrigley, *Poverty, Progress, and Population*, p. 90.
19. R. Wood, *The Population of Britain in the Nineteenth Century* (London: Macmillan, 1992), p. 25
20. P. Clark, 'Introduction,' in J. Stobart and P. Lane (eds.), *Urban and Industrial Change in the Midlands 1700–1840* (Leicester: Centre for Urban History, 2000).
21. J. Langton, 'Town Growth and Urbanisation in the Midlands from the 1660s to 1841,' in Stobart and Lane (eds.), *Urban and Industrial Change in the Midlands 1700–1840* (Leicester: Centre for Urban History, 2000).
22. Roger Scola, *Feeding the Victorian City: The Food Supply of Manchester, 1770–1870* (Manchester: Manchester University Press, 1992), pp. 17–19.
23. Claire Townsend, 'County versus Region? Migrational Connections in the East Midlands, 1700–1830,' *Journal of Historical Geography*, 32/2 (2006), pp. 291–312.
24. Wood, *Population of Britain*, p. 28.
25. Scull, *Museums of Madness.*
26. Wrigley, *Poverty, Progress, and Population*, pp. 107–108.
27. 'Insanity and Agricultural Depression,' *BMJ*, 1881, 1/1053, p. 351.
28. J. Stobart, *The First Industrial Region: North-West England, c.1700–60* (Manchester: Manchester University Press, 2004), p. 10.

29. C. Pooley, 'The Influence of Locality on Migration: A Comparative Study of Britain and Sweden in the Nineteenth Century,' *Local Population Studies*, 90/1 (2013), pp. 13–27.
30. Barrie Trinder, 'Towns and Industries: The Changing Character of Manufacturing Towns,' in Stobart and Raven, *Towns, Regions and Industries*, pp. 102–120, p. 113; Ron Greenall, *A History of Northamptonshire and the Soke of Peterborough* (Chichester: Phillimore, 2000), pp. 114–116.
31. Greenall, *Northamptonshire*, p. 114; Trinder, 'Towns and industries,' p. 113.
32. *Northampton Mercury*, 22 December 1883, p. 6.
33. *Northampton Mercury*, 27 February 1891, p. 2.
34. *Bucks Herald*, 8 February 1873, p. 4.
35. *Bucks Herald*, 16 November 1872, p. 4.
36. *Bucks Herald*, 8 February 1873, p. 4.
37. Trinder, 'Towns and Industries,' p. 114.
38. *Northampton Mercury*, 29 December 1899, p. 7.
39. *Northampton Mercury*, 29 December 1899, p. 7.
40. *Northampton Mercury*, 22 December 1883, p. 6.
41. M. Hanly, 'The Economy of Makeshifts and the Role of the Poor Law: A Game of Chance?,' in S. King and A. Tomkins (eds.), *The Poor in England 1700–1850: An Economy* 2003), pp. 76–99, p. 77.
42. Greenall, *Northamptonshire*, p. 119.
43. C. Cox et al., 'Emaciated, Exhausted and Excited'.
44. GMCRO, Lancashire Asylums Board Processdings, 29 November 1894, A/Pres, pp. 11–12.
45. W.A.F. Browne, 'What Asylums Were, Are, and Ought to be,' in A. Scull (ed.), *The Asylum as Utopia: W.A.F Browne and the Mid-Nineteenth Century Consolidation of Psychiatry* (London: Routledge, 1991), p. 58; J. Bucknill and D.H. Tuke, *A Manual of Psychological Medicine: Containing the History, Nosology, Description, Statistics, Diagnosis, Pathology and Treatment of Insanity* (London: John Churchill, 1858).
46. E.F. Torrey, *Schizophrenia and Civilisation* (New York: Jason Aronson, 1980); E. Hare, 'Was Insanity on the Increase?,' *British Journal of Psychiatry*, 142/4 (1983), 439–455; E. Hare, 'Aspects of the Epidemiology of Schizophrenia,' *British Journal of Psychiatry*, 149 (1986), pp. 554–561.
47. Melling, 'Proper Lunatic'.
48. LMA, Friern Hospital (Colney Hatch), Male Casebook 6, H12/CH/B/13/006, William Langley, Admission no. 1746.
49. Melling et al., 'Proper Lunatic,' p. 374. In Devon there were 101 children identified that were admitted to the asylum. However, these figures

included 23 children that were aged fourteen. In order to make an accurate comparison these 23 children were not included in the calculation.

50. Wright, *Earlswood*, chap. 3; Wright, 'Familial Care of "Idiot" Children in Victorian England,' in P. Horden and R. Smith, *The Locus of Care: Families, Communities, Institutions, and the Provisions of Welfare since Antiquity* (London: Routledge, 1998), pp. 176–197.
51. Smith, 'Living with Insanity'.
52. V. Skultans, *English Madness: Ideas on Insanity, 1580–1890* (London: Routledge, 1979), p. 7.
53. BLAS, Three Counties Asylum, Male Patient Casebook 2, LF31/2, p. 140.
54. LRO, Prestiwch Asylum, Male Patient Casebook 6, QAM6/6/6, Brocklehurst.
55. C.H. Lee, 'Regional Inequalities in Infant Mortality in Britain, 1861–1971: Patterns and Hypotheses,' *Population Studies*, 45/1 (1991), pp. 55–65, p. 63.
56. H. Newton, 'Children's Physic: Medical Perceptions and Treatment of Sick Children in Early Modern England,' *Social History of Medicine*, 23/3 (2010), pp. 456–474, p. 461; H. Newton, *The Sick Child in Early Modern England* (Oxford: Oxford University Press, 2012).
57. A. Borsay, *Disability and Social Policy in Britain Since 1750* (Basingstoke: Palgrave Macmillan, 2005), p. 74; Also, Digby on the size and evolution of the Retreat, *Madness, Morality and Medicine: A Study of the York Retreat, 1796–1914* (Cambridge: Cambridge University Press, 1985).
58. P. Bartlett, *The Poor Law of Lunacy: The Administration of Pauper Lunatics in Mid-Nineteenth-Century England* (London: Leicester University Press, 1999); P. Bartlett, 'The Asylum and the Poor Law: The Productive Alliance,' in J. Melling and B. Forsythe (eds.), *Insanity, Institutions and Society, 1800–1914: A Social History of Madness in Comparative Perspective* (London: Routledge, 1999), pp. 48–67; D.M. Jones, 'The Custody and Care of the Mentally Ill in Lancashire—Historical Perspectives and Sources,' in J.V. Pickstone (ed.), *Health, Disease and Medicine in Lancashire 1750–1950* (Manchester: North West Community Newspapers Limited, 1980), pp. 66–86.
59. J.F. Saunders, *Institutionalised Offenders—A Study of the Victorian Institution and its Inmates, with Special Reference to Late Nineteenth Century Warwickshire* (University of Warwick: Unpublished PhD Thesis, 1983), pp. 137–154.
60. NRO, St Crispin Collection, Male Casebook, NCLA/6/2/2/5, Arthur Hillam, Admission no. 2725, p. 229; NRO, St Crispin Collection, Out of County Casebook 1, NCLA/6/2/3/1, Thomas Thomas, Admission no.

2842, p. 250; NRO, St Crispin Collection, Out of County Casebook 1, NCLA/6/2/3/1, Jane Ball, p. 618.

61. BLA, Three Counties, Female Casebook 9, LF29/9, Elizabeth Mead, Admission no. 5434, p. 194; BLA, Three Counties, Female Casebook 9, LF29/9, Mary Ann Pilgrim, Admission no. 5198, p. 80; BLA, Three Counties, Male Casebook 2, LF31/2, Sidney Woodland, Admission no. 1795, p. 227.
62. M. Archer, *Idiocy and Institutionalisation in Late Victorian Britain. The Warwick County Idiot Asylum 1852 to 1877* (University of Warwick: Unpublished MA Thesis, 2010).
63. BLA, Three Counties, Male Casebook 7, LF31/7, William Clarvis, Admission no. 4595, p. 199.
64. BLA, Three Counties, Male Casebook 6, LF31/6, Samuel Parrish, Admission no. 3966, p. 144; BLA, Three Counties, Female Casebook 7, LF29/7, Kate Chapman, Admission no. 8277, p. 175.
65. BCA, All Saints, Male Casebook 13, MS344/12/13, Thomas Skirrow, Admission no. 8621, pp. 429–430.
66. NRO, St Crispin Collection, Female Casebook 5, NCLA/6/2/1/5, Caroline Clements, Admission no. 1927, p. 35.
67. BLA, Three Counties, Male Casebook 5, LF31/5, George Clark, Admission no. 3186.
68. Melling, 'Proper Lunatic'.

CHAPTER 4

Looking Out from the Asylum: Deathbeds, Distribution, and Diversity

Up until this point the focus has been on the 'insane' child and their experiences of confinement inside the asylum. Now we begin to explore the role of the institution in a wider economy of care for mentally impaired children, and ask if it pulled in youngsters from around a network of welfare or whether it acted as a carousel to circulate children through a system of alternative provision. The function of asylums in any 'mixed economy' of care that may have existed was thought to have been ended by the prescriptive lunacy legislation of 1845.[1] After this watershed historians have assumed that the only alternatives for managing the health and behaviour of the insane occurred in the workhouse or domestic and community spheres.[2] Consequently, discussions about caring for the insane in the second half of the nineteenth century are restricted to asylums, homes, and workhouses.[3] Even in the rare instances when the literature has extended its analysis beyond the asylum it has failed to include the experience of children. Therefore it is important to locate the asylum, as an institution of care for the young, in a broader landscape of provision for both the poor and the sick.

To do so this chapter will be broken down into three sections. The first explores the social spaces from where children were sent to the asylum and, developing the discussion of the previous chapter, the institutional places that they were subsequently discharged to, if they were lucky enough to leave. This locates children's movements through the system of welfare and traces their journeys between institutions. Secondly, the

S.J. Taylor, *Child Insanity in England, 1845-1907*, Palgrave Studies in the History of Childhood, DOI 10.1007/978-1-137-60027-1_4

analysis will be expanded to reconsider the nature of our asylums by locality. It will explore the differing approaches of each institution and further demonstrate how their management was affected by regional and local concerns. An exploration of relationships between the Poor Law and asylum will be crucial, especially in the Lancashire region. The final section examines intra-regional Poor Law attitudes towards the asylum in Northamptonshire and extends the discussion of the complex local politics that affected admissions.

The Mixed Economy of Care

Asylums have been viewed in a variety of ways, from institutions of control and regulation to hospices for the care of the terminally ill.[4] But any comprehension of their role in a broader economy of medical care has been overlooked. Children, we can observe, were admitted to asylums from numerous places and spaces (Table 4.1). We have already seen that the ethos of the Northamptonshire institution meant that it had the largest percentage of children admitted from other asylums. And, as might be expected, Colney Hatch, due to its proximity to the metropolis, had the most routes into the asylum, but it is difficult to assess whether this was a trend for all urban institutions due to incomplete datasets. In Manchester the number of unknown cases might be indicative of broader attitudes towards child patients; children were seen as inferior and, in line with the causative framework already established, it was not deemed important to record all of their information. The percentage of unknown cases was also high for the Birmingham Asylum because some of the records for the asylum are unfit for public viewing due to fire and flood damage.

There are clearly difficulties in building detailed pictures of where children were admitted from in the case of urban asylums. These places were regularly not recorded and thus complicate any attempt at compiling individual histories. For example, George Clift was admitted to Birmingham at the age of four in 1881, his case history for the period of confinement is complete with the one omission of where he was sent to the asylum from.[5] Similarly, at Colney Hatch, Susan Squires was admitted as an imbecile, aged eleven, in 1858.[6] Her casefile records that she was of weak intellect, but fails to reveal whether she was previously resident in the family home, workhouse, or a different place of care. The information from rural institutions is more complete but routes to the asylum were less diverse in these areas. In accordance with current historiographical thinking, the

Table 4.1 Locations from where children were admitted to the asylum

	Asylum (in county)	*Asylum (out county)*	*Home*	*Hospital*	*Idiot Asylum*	*Private Institution*	*School*	*Workhouse (inc. lunatic wards)*	*Unknown*
Birmingham	0	6 (6%)	24 (25%)	1 (1%)	0	0	0	20 (21%)	44 (46%)
Colney Hatch	9 (4%)	13 (6%)	88 (41%)	1 (0.4%)	4 (2%)	1 (0.4%)	1 (0.4%)	50 (23%)	46 (22%)
Manchester	2 (3%)	0	15 (21%)	0	0	0	0	8 (11%)	47 (65%)
Northampton	0	61 (27%)	142 (62%)	0	0	0	1 (0.4%)	16 (7%)	9 (4%)
Three Counties	2 (1%)	2 (1%)	98 (60%)	0	0	0	1 (0.6%)	30 (19%)	31 (19%)
Total	13 (2%)	82 (10%)	367 (48%)	2 (<1%)	4 (<1%)	1 (<1%)	3 (<1%)	124 (16%)	177 (23%)

Source: BCL, Male Patient Casebooks, MS344/12/2 & 2a, MS344/12/5, MS344/12/7-9, MS344/12/11-14, MS344/12/20-22, MS344/12/27; BCL, Female Patient Casebooks, MS344/12/41-47, MS344/12/49-51, MS344/12/53 & 54, MS344/12/56 & 57, MS344/12/60-63; BCL, Patient Index, MS344/11/1 & 2; LMA, Colney Hatch Male Patient Casebooks, H12/CH/B/13/001-61; LMA, Colney Hatch Female Patient Casebooks, H12/CH/B/11/001-085; NRO, Male Patient Casebooks, NCLA/6/2/2/1-12; NRO Female Patient Casebooks, NCLA/6/2/1/1-13; GMCRO, Male Patient Casebooks, ADMM/2/1-16; GMCRO, ADMF/2/1-21; LRO, Male Patient Casebooks, QAM/6/6/1-34; LRO, Female Patient Casebooks, QAM/6/6/1-34; BLAS, Male Patient Casebooks, LF31/1-12; BLAS, Female Patient Casebooks, LF29/1-1

home was the most common destination from which children were dispatched to the asylum, followed by the workhouse in these areas.

The image remains ambiguous if the focus is shifted towards how children departed asylums. For example, some were discharged as 'recovered' but their destinations upon leaving the asylum are unclear. A case in point is that of John Feltham who was sent to Colney Hatch from the Islington Workhouse, aged thirteen.[7] After spending six weeks in the asylum he had recovered from his bout of mania and was discharged on 3 August 1883. In this situation there is no information as to where Feltham went after leaving Colney Hatch. Feltham's case is emblematic of all of those discharged as recovered with the exception of one boy. It was noted on the casefile of Thomas Walker that upon recovery he was returned to his mother, after spending two years inside Colney Hatch.[8] Until it is revealed otherwise, it will have to be assumed that those who had recovered returned to the domestic sphere. This is because the involvement of the Poor Law was usually explicitly mentioned in other departures and led to the reason for discharge being recorded as 'relieved', rather than 'recovered'—a statement about the withdrawal of funding from Guardians instead of a comment on the improvement of a child's mental health. Further problems are posed by those with casefiles that ended abruptly with no clue as to their future destinations. In these situations there may have been no information recorded about the child's departure or patient data may have extended into continuation books that are currently embargoed by the Data Protection Act. These issues notwithstanding, the fundamental typological differences between rural and urban institutions are reinforced by the patterns of discharge presented in Table 4.2. The numbers, whilst at times small, exemplify the variations that existed between the different 'types' of asylums examined. We know that death rates in rural asylums were high but it is startling how few children managed to leave these institutions. Urban asylums on the other hand had access to a wider range of options and could move individuals with more ease.[9]

The contrasts between the rural and urban are better visualised in the form of a flow diagram (Fig. 4.1). In this format it is evident that the asylum in the rural location captured large numbers of children and that the urban distributed them around a network of care. A number of emblematic case studies embody these institutional experiences. Alfred Morran was diagnosed as an idiot and transferred to Colney Hatch from the Fisherton House Asylum in Wiltshire on 21 July 1871. Prior to being sent to Fisherton House he had been an inmate of the Clerkenwell Workhouse

Table 4.2 Discharge data by asylum

	Asylum (in County)	*Asylum (out of County)*	*Died*	*Parents/Friends*	*Hospital*	*School*	*Workhouse*	*Unknown*
Birmingham	13 (14%)	4 (4%)	16 (17%)	36 (38%)	0	0	4 (4%)	22 (23%)
Colney Hatch	11 (5%)	3 (1%)	85 (40%)	50 (23%)	0	12 (6%)	53 (25%)	0
Manchester	33 (46%)	0	7 (10%)	14 (19%)	0	0	15 (21%)	3 (4%)
Northampton	0	31 (13%)	135 (58%)	27 (12%)	1 (0.4%)	0	25 (11%)	12 (5%)
Three Counties	0	17 (11%)	108 (67%)	32 (20%)	0	0	3 (2%)	1 (0.6%)

Source: BCL, Male Patient Casebooks, MS344/12/2 & 2a, MS344/12/5, MS344/12/7-9, MS344/12/11-14, MS344/12/20-22, MS344/12/27; BCL, Female Patient Casebooks, MS344/12/41-47, MS344/12/49-51, MS344/12/53 & 54, MS344/12/56 & 57, MS344/12/60-63; BCL, Patient Index, MS344/11/1 & 2; LMA, Colney Hatch Male Patient Casebooks, H12/CH/B/13/001-61; LMA, Colney Hatch Female Patient Casebooks, H12/CH/B/11/001-085; NRO, Male Patient Casebooks, NCLA/6/2/2/1-12; NRO Female Patient Casebooks, NCLA/6/2/1/1-13; GMCRO, Male Patient Casebooks, ADMM/2/1-16; GMRCO, ADMF/2/1-21; LRO, Male Patient Casebooks, QAM/6/6/1-34; LRO, Female Patient Casebooks, QAM/6/6/1-34; BLAS, Male Patient Casebooks, LF31/1-12; BLAS, Female Patient Casebooks, LF29/1-12

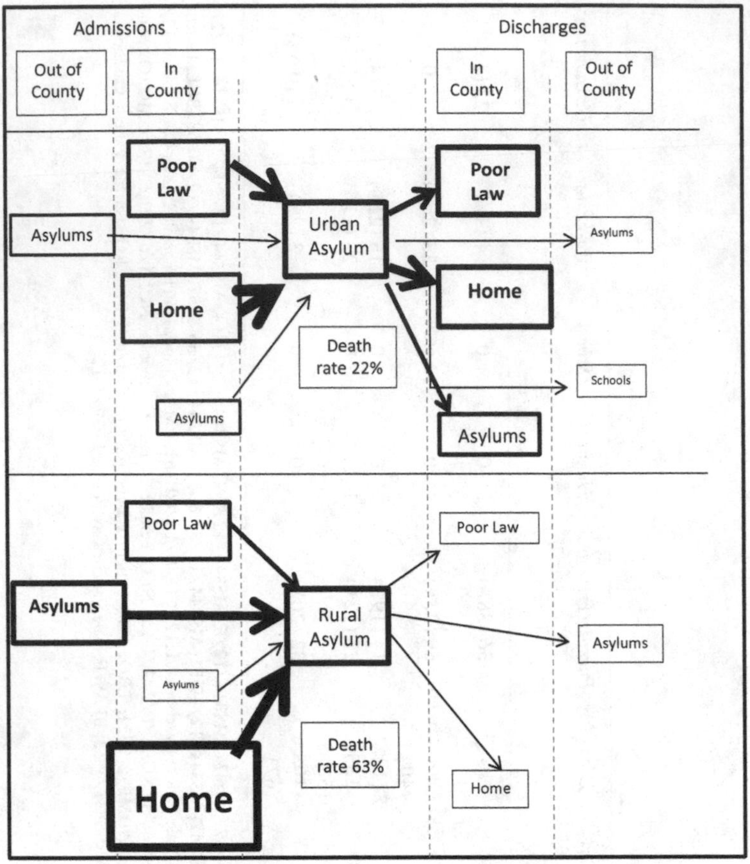

Fig. 4.1 Flow chart of admissions and discharges to urban and rural asylums. (Box and arrow size are tuned to quantity; the bigger the box the more children were coming from or going to that location). *Source*: BCL, Male Patient Casebooks, MS344/12/2 & 2a, MS344/12/5, MS344/12/7-9, MS344/12/11-14, MS344/12/20-22, MS344/12/27; BCL, Female Patient Casebooks, MS344/12/41-47, MS344/12/49-51, MS344/12/53 & 54, MS344/12/56 & 57, MS344/12/60-63; BCL, Patient Index, MS344/11/1 & 2; LMA, Colney Hatch Male Patient Casebooks, H12/CH/B/13/001-61; LMA, Colney Hatch Female Patient Casebooks, H12/CH/B/11/001-085; NRO, Male Patient Casebooks, NCLA/6/2/2/1-12; NRO Female Patient Casebooks, NCLA/6/2/1/1-13; GMCRO, Male Patient Casebooks, ADMM/2/1-16; GMRCO, ADMF/2/1-21; LRO, Male Patient Casebooks, QAM/6/6/1-34; LRO, Female Patient Casebooks, QAM/6/6/1-34; BLAS, Male Patient Casebooks, LF31/1-12; BLAS, Female Patient Casebooks, LF29/1-12

for two and a half years. After spending just over eighteen months at Colney Hatch he was transferred to the Caterham Asylum for idiots, completing quite an extensive tour of institutional confinement.[10] Alfred Sowter, who featured in Chap. 2 and was described as dangerous after trying to kill his mother, was admitted to the Colney Hatch Asylum on 13 February 1897. He had been admitted from the Wandsworth Poor Law Union infirmary where he was diagnosed as an imbecile. He remained in the asylum for just over a month before being discharged to the Darenth Schools in Kent.[11] At the Birmingham asylum, Maria Butler was admitted from the Aston Workhouse on 22 July 1882 and fifteen months later was transferred to the Rubery Hill Asylum on the outskirts of the city.[12] When the Prestwich Asylum was opened in 1851 Edward Ridings was admitted from the Haydock Lodge Asylum. A year later he was moved out of Prestwich to the Oldham Workhouse.[13] These children demonstrate how urban asylums acted as clearing houses for those with mental illnesses and disabilities. By fulfilling this function the institution provided a particular response to this type of patient that aided it in tackling wider institutional issues such as overcrowding.

Unsurprisingly, experiences in the rural asylum were the polar opposite. At the Three Counties Asylum John Beale, aged thirteen, was admitted in 1867 and confined until he died 28 years later.[14] Also at Three Counties, Edwin Seabrook was confined for thirty-five years, John Prutton for thirty-nine years, Alfred Lester for thirty-one years, Ada Harding for thirty-three years, and Henry Aylett for thirty years, all of whom died inside the institution.[15] The picture was similar in the Berrywood Asylum, where Charles York, Joseph Harris, Lucy Jones and Elizabeth Robinson were all confined for over thirty years.[16] The most extreme example of the rural asylum holding onto child patients is provided by Priscilla Elliot, who was admitted at the age of eight to Three Counties Asylum. She was diagnosed as an imbecile and remained in the asylum for the rest of her life, an astonishing fifty-four years.[17]

The Rubery Hill Asylum in Birmingham, 'the Annex' at Prestwich in Manchester, and the Metropolitan Asylum Board institutions of Leavesden and Caterham Imbecile Asylums as well as the Darenth School, all represented efforts to offer institutional space for patients that did not fit with the curative goals of pauper lunatic asylums in urban areas. These spaces of care were all created from the late-1860s when it was evident that the number of pauper lunatics exceeded the room available in asylums. By developing extra capacity for the chronic and harmless, it was thought that asylums could be cleared to make room for curable patients and those suffering acute disorders. Their importance to the larger county lunatic asylums has therefore been overlooked by historians. David Wright has argued that the creation of extra asylum space marked a change in the care provided for those with learning disabilities by the state. He, however, suggests that this was only the case for London where there was 'a veritable musical chairs of institutional provision for the learning disabled and the mentally ill'.[18] The asylums located in Birmingham and Manchester demonstrated that provision for chronic and harmless patients was developed in urban areas outside of the capital during the late-nineteenth century. In contrast, areas served by rural asylums continued with the traditional coping mechanisms of the workhouse and community.

When discussing the children that were either circulated out of urban institutions or retained in rural asylums it is important to investigate the patients that did not conform to 'type'. In other words, those that were not circulated from urban asylums to other provision, the 22 % that died. Why did they not get moved on to other asylums, workhouses, or back home to parents or families? Also what distinguished the 27 % of children that were pulled into the rural institution but were then circulated to other provision? To understand the asylum system and its carousel it is crucial to understand the way that these institutions filtered their child patients.

Confinement and Circulation

The manner in which patients moved through systems of welfare in the nineteenth century is an under-researched topic.[19] By better understanding the way that people moved between medical institutions in the nineteenth century it is possible to reveal attitudes towards children and demonstrate how a medical economy of makeshifts operated. Through the prism of child patients it is possible to explore the experiences of circulation or retention in the broader networks of medical care that existed. Looking firstly at urban asylums, boys made up 66 % of those admitted and they were also disproportionately less likely to be circulated to alternative provision. They accounted for 75 % of child patient deaths inside these institutions. Developing the picture further, Fig. 4.2 demonstrates that older children at admission were more likely to die in urban asylums, although we already know that they were also the most likely to be admitted. Considering the sample through a more medical lens, 29 % of the children not circulated had causative explanations for their conditions; this corresponds with the overall figure of urban asylums providing causes for

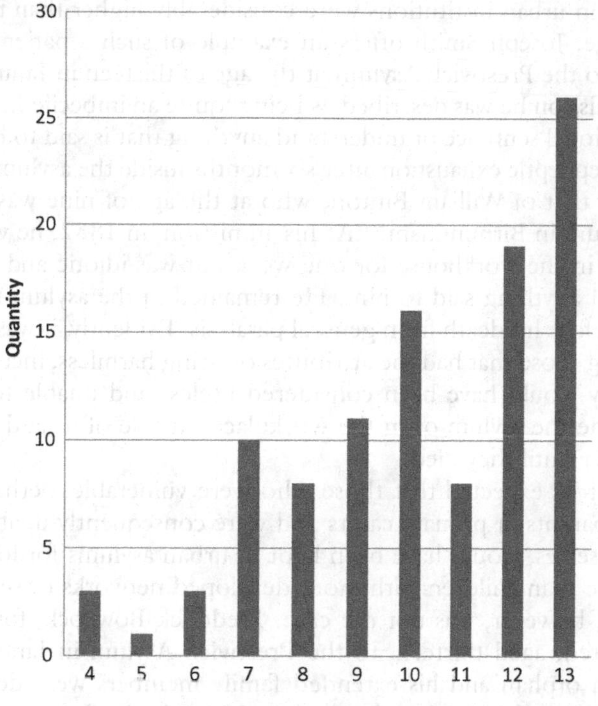

Fig. 4.2 Age at admission of children that died in urban asylums. *Source*: BCL, Male Patient Casebooks, MS344/12/2 & 2a, MS344/12/5, MS344/12/7-9, MS344/12/11-14, MS344/12/20-22, MS344/12/27; BCL, Female Patient Casebooks, MS344/12/41-47, MS344/12/49-51, MS344/12/53 & 54, MS344/12/56 & 57, MS344/12/60-63; BCL, Patient Index, MS344/11/1 & 2; LMA, Colney Hatch Male Patient Casebooks, H12/CH/B/13/001-61; LMA, Colney Hatch Female Patient Casebooks, H12/CH/B/11/001-085; NRO, Male Patient Casebooks, NCLA/6/2/2/1-12; NRO Female Patient Casebooks, NCLA/6/2/1/1-13; GMCRO, Male Patient Casebooks, ADMM/2/1-16; GMCRO, ADMF/2/1-21; LRO, Male Patient Casebooks, QAM/6/6/1-34; LRO, Female Patient Casebooks, QAM/6/6/1-34; BLAS, Male Patient Casebooks, LF31/1-12; BLAS, Female Patient Casebooks, LF29/1-12

30 % of all child cases. Thus it appears that causality did not stand out as a factor in circulation. The diagnosis, however, was more significant. Those retained were most commonly classified as idiots or imbeciles (87%), with mania (8%), dementia (4%) and general paralysis (1%) accounting for the remaining diagnoses. Instances of mental disability amongst those kept

long term in urban institutions were considerably higher than the collective average. Joseph Smith offers an example of such a patient. He was admitted to the Prestwich Asylum at the age of thirteen in January 1890. Upon admission he was described as being 'quite an imbecile … unable to speak a rational sentence or understand anything that is said to him'.[20] He died from epileptic exhaustion after six months inside the asylum. Another example is that of William Binton, who at the age of nine was admitted to the asylum in Birmingham.[21] At his admission, in 1882, he was said to have been in the workhouse for one week but was idiotic and could not understand anything said to him. He remained in the asylum for almost six years before his death from general paralysis. Evidently, it was harder to move along those that had the attributes of being harmless, incurable, and male. They would have been considered useless and unable to improve either inside the asylum or in the workplace outside of it, and were thus left to fester until they died.

It might be expected that those who were vulnerable, perhaps having lost their parents or primary carers and were consequently unable to look after themselves, would have been kept in urban asylums for longer periods of time than children with more developed networks of support and care. This, however, was not the case. Frederick Bowcock, for example, was admitted, aged thirteen, to the Prestwich Asylum in January 1881. He was an orphan and his extended family members were described as 'intemperate' and were therefore unsuitable to look after a mentally disabled child.[22] Notwithstanding his lack of parents and potentially deviant family, Bowcock was discharged four months after admission described as recovered. It is unclear whether he went to live with his intemperate family or elsewhere.

By continuing to focus on those that were not circulated from urban asylums, it could be assumed that the 22 % of children retained simply died after spending a short amount of time there. This was certainly true for a small number of cases. James Gray was only a patient at Colney Hatch for fourteen days before he died.[23] But, his example was not a common experience and the average length of confinement for those retained in urban asylums was seven years and five months. The longest amount of time spent inside an urban institution by a child patient was at Colney Hatch, where Mary Ann Beard remained twenty-four years and eleven months.[24] Such an experience was more in line with that of rural asylums, demonstrating the similar regulatory roles that institutions could provide for those that had limited chances of improvement.

In rural areas the characteristics of children circulated to and from asylums are significant when establishing how a mixed economy of care operated. In total there were 105 (27%) children that came to rural asylums from other institutions. These locations were asylums, schools or workhouses. Of these, fifty-two died and the remainder were circulated to the following destinations: twenty-six to other asylums, five relieved to Poor Law Unions, nineteen recovered and three had incomplete case records. In total just under a third were circulated back to other institutional settings. While this figure might appear low, children admitted from institutional care accounted for 54 % of all transfers out of the rural asylum to other institutional provision. Movement between institutions of care and welfare was a feature of the rural asylum even if it was on a smaller scale than in large industrial cities. Therefore some similarity in the function of urban and rural asylums can be observed.

Looking at all admissions to rural asylums, there were 24 % of children that left as recovered. The remainder were circulated still suffering from the afflictions, illnesses, and disabilities that led to their confinement. Only 10 % of these were sent back to Poor Law Guardians. The discharge of children to the Poor Law usually came at the request of the Board of Guardians who were no longer willing to pay the fees for the asylum. Yet, the number of children that departed in this way was small and suggests that cost was not an important factor in removal for most cases. If those that were reclaimed by the Poor Law are omitted, 24 % of all child admissions were moved out of asylums in rural areas.

Unlike their urban counterparts, gender was not a determining factor in the selection process of who was moved out of rural asylums. The cohort of children circulated was made up of 59 % male and 41 % female patients. This is a close reflection of all the child patients which was made up of 60 % male and 40 % female. In the previous chapter it was observed that the age distribution of children at admission to rural asylums was much smoother than for urban asylums. From Fig. 4.3 it can be observed that countryside children, much like in urban institutions, were more likely to be moved out of rural asylums if they were older when admitted. The children themselves can provide an explanation for this similarity; through prolonged confinement younger patients became institutionalised and when employed around the asylum were an economic asset to the institution and were thus worth holding on to.

The children that were circulated from rural institutions, however, usually spent significant amounts of time there. Those that were discharged

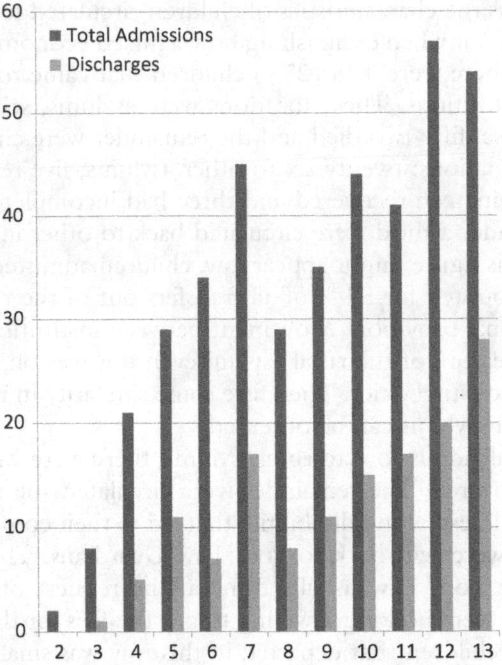

Fig. 4.3 Rates of discharge by age at admission for rural asylums. The total number of discharges was 140. *Source*: BCL, Male Patient Casebooks, MS344/12/2 & 2a, MS344/12/5, MS344/12/7-9, MS344/12/11-14, MS344/12/20-22, MS344/12/27; BCL, Female Patient Casebooks, MS344/12/41-47, MS344/12/49-51, MS344/12/53 & 54, MS344/12/56 & 57, MS344/12/60-63; BCL, Patient Index, MS344/11/1 & 2; LMA, Colney Hatch Male Patient Casebooks, H12/CH/B/13/001-61; LMA, Colney Hatch Female Patient Casebooks, H12/CH/B/11/001-085; NRO, Male Patient Casebooks, NCLA/6/2/2/1-12; NRO Female Patient Casebooks, NCLA/6/2/1/1-13; GMCRO, Male Patient Casebooks, ADMM/2/1-16; GMCRO, ADMF/2/1-21; LRO, Male Patient Casebooks, QAM/6/6/1-34; LRO, Female Patient Casebooks, QAM/6/6/1-34; BLAS, Male Patient Casebooks, LF31/1-12; BLAS, Female Patient Casebooks, LF29/1-12

as recovered were confined on average for just under two years and two months, but children that were moved to Poor Law Guardians or parents and friends that had not recovered stayed in the asylum on average for five years and seven months. And children that were moved to alternative provision, and thus remained in the economy of care, stayed in the asylum seven years and six months on average. Even though older children were the most likely to move on from rural asylums, they still spent significant amounts of time confined and circulation did not operate in the same way as it did in urban areas.

It has been suggested that rural institutions were more thorough in their causative assessments of child insanity. To revisit that analysis, a causative explanation was provided in 46 % of rural cases. Considering how these children fit in a mixed economy of rural care provides an insight into the medical nature and character of these institutions. Looking at those that were discharged reveals that 53 % of them had a causative explanation for their condition. A closer examination of these children shows that 29 % recovered, 11 % returned to families not improved, and 7 % were discharged as not improved but without a recorded destination. The remainder were kept in a mixed economy of care with 39 % transferred to other asylums and 14 % to Poor Law Guardians. The children circulated to other provision were diagnosed predominantly with learning disabilities (79 % were recorded as idiots, 13 % as imbeciles, 4 % demented and 4 % as dumb and paralysed). The causative explanations were mostly hereditary, accounting for 75 %, acquired causes accounting for 17 %, and developmental 8 %. It can be argued that the diagnostic investigation in the case of these children meant they remained in the economy of care for longer. The average length of confinement for them, before being circulated to alternative arrangements, was nineteen years and two months. The dominance of hereditary causes, linked to the increased influence of eugenicist ideas, implies that most of the children circulated were admitted to the asylum from the 1880s onwards. Figure 4.4 confirms this, with all hereditary causes being admitted to the rural asylum after 1885.

Such long durations of confinement for children suggest that the rural asylum was a magnet for child patients. The majority were only circulated in the wake of legislative changes introduced by the School Medical Service in 1907. These required Local Education Authorities to provide treatment for those with special educational needs. After 1907 those remaining in asylums were removed at the outbreak of war in 1914 when some asylums were used for the treatment and recuperation of soldiers

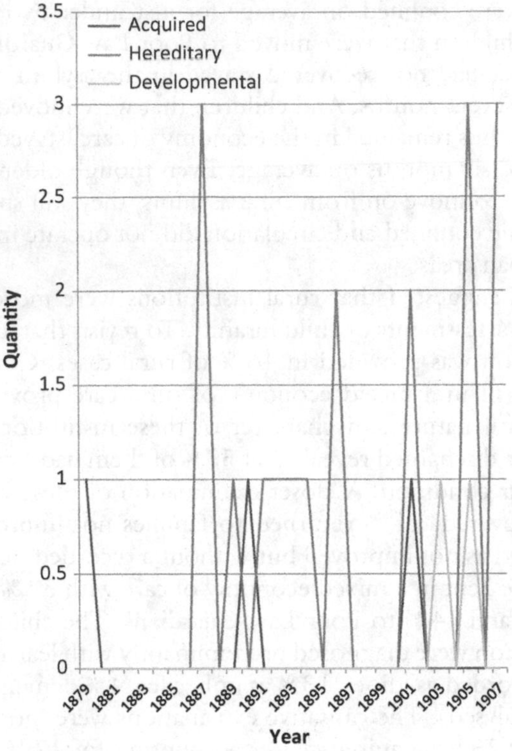

Fig. 4.4 Causative explanations for children remaining in the mixed economy of care. *Source*: BCL, Male Patient Casebooks, MS344/12/2 & 2a, MS344/12/5, MS344/12/7-9, MS344/12/11-14, MS344/12/20-22, MS344/12/27; BCL, Female Patient Casebooks, MS344/12/41-47, MS344/12/49-51, MS344/12/53 & 54, MS344/12/56 & 57, MS344/12/60-63; BCL, Patient Index, MS344/11/1 & 2; LMA, Colney Hatch Male Patient Casebooks, H12/CH/B/13/001-61; LMA, Colney Hatch Female Patient Casebooks, H12/CH/B/11/001-085; NRO, Male Patient Casebooks, NCLA/6/2/2/1-12; NRO Female Patient Casebooks, NCLA/6/2/1/1-13; GMCRO, Male Patient Casebooks, ADMM/2/1-16; GMCRO, ADMF/2/1-21; LRO, Male Patient Casebooks, QAM/6/6/1-34; LRO, Female Patient Casebooks, QAM/6/6/1-34; BLAS, Male Patient Casebooks, LF31/1-12; BLAS, Female Patient Casebooks, LF29/1-12

from the frontline. The impact of these events is evident from Fig. 4.5. Consequently, it is difficult to identify a model child that was circulated from the rural asylums. What can be noted is that children entering rural institutions often spent the rest of their lives there and if they did leave it was most likely to be transferred to a different institution. Even when those admitted as children did manage to leave the asylum they remained confined for extended periods of time.

Identifying Systems of Care

The most obvious alternative space for the care of the pauper insane during the period was the Poor Law workhouse. However, when the relationship between the Poor Law system and asylums has been assessed by historians, it has been analysed from a top-down and policy driven perspective that only features the individual experience in a generic and

Fig 4.5 Years of departure for children with causative explanations. *Source*: NRO, Male Patient Casebooks, NCLA/6/2/2/1-12; NRO Female Patient Casebooks, NCLA/6/2/1/1-13; BLAS, Male Patient Casebooks, LF31/1-12; BLAS, Female Patient Casebooks, LF29/1-12

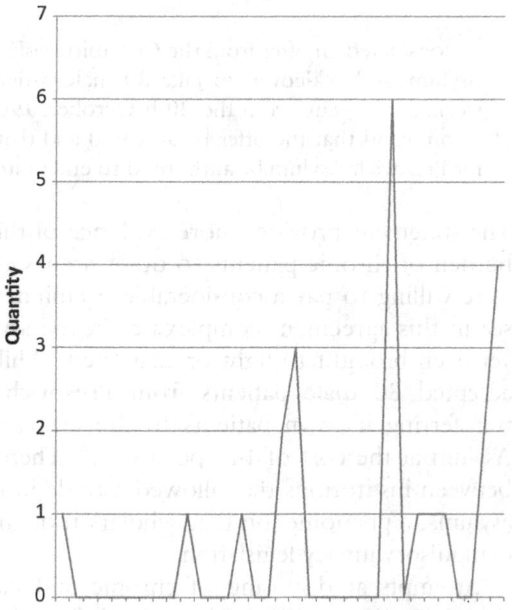

fleeting fashion. A consequence of such an approach is that within the current literature there is limited consideration of the variations in patient populations and experiences, and regions are considered in isolation with a failure to compare and contrast the wider picture.[25] Moving forward the challenge is to rectify some of these problems. The incurability of chronic and harmless child asylum patients meant that they posed particular problems to the institutions that confined them.[26] In 1894 the Prestwich Asylum, in an effort to alleviate the burden that these cases placed on space, came to an agreement with the Rochdale Poor Law Union to send eighty harmless incurables to their workhouse infirmary.[27] Such an agreement is further evidence of the divergent approaches of the five asylums. The Prestwich Asylum circulated patients around the system of welfare, displaying the willingness of this particular institution to use workhouses to accommodate those deemed harmless. In contrast, Northampton was eager to attract child patients to its asylum from all over the country in order to boost its profits.[28] The agreement with Rochdale was not the only arrangement put in place to deal with chronic and harmless children. In 1900 the Lancashire Asylums Board:

> … considered an offer from the Committee of Visitors of the Derby County Asylum, at Mickleover, to take 30 male patients for the sum of 16*s*. per week, per patient, from the 20th October, 1900. Your Committee beg to recommend that the offer be accepted and that the Committee of Visitors for Prestwich Asylum be authorised to enter into the necessary agreement.[29]

The statement provides more evidence of the urban asylum shifting the burden of chronic patients to other arenas of care. In this instance they were willing to pay a considerable premium in order to do so. We thus see in this agreement complexities in the asylum network that have not yet been brought to light or examined. While the asylum at Mickleover accepted 30 male patients from Prestwich, the same institution was transferring its own patients to the entrepreneurial Northamptonshire Asylum at the cost of 14*s*. per week.[30] There was an interconnectedness between institutions that allowed a trade in the insane during the era of asylums, a phenomenon that scholars thought ended with the passing of compulsory lunacy legislation.

Attempts at disposing of chronic and harmless patients from overcrowded urban asylums always had financial incentives attached. They either took the form of increased premiums or additional payments to Poor

Law Guardians. During the late 1890s when asylum space in Lancashire was most sought after, the Lancashire Asylums Board (LAB) offered Poor Law Unions in the county an extension of the 4*s*. grant for every chronic patient, certified as insane, that was confined in a workhouse rather than an asylum. In 1895 the Lancashire Asylums Board declared:

> That, as it is not desirable that idiots should be treated in a Lunatic Asylum, the 4s. grants shall, wherever idiots are kept at the public expense, be payable in regard to such idiots to the Authority maintaining them to the satisfaction of the Commissioners in Lunacy. A certificate by any authority prescribed by the Local Government Board shall be a sufficient title to the grant aforesaid.[31]

It had been assumed that this grant had the effect of clogging up workhouses with chronic and harmless patients discharged from asylums.[32] But revisionist historians have shown that its impact was minimal.[33] Such an effort by the LAB was an attempt to convince Poor Law Guardians to divert the burden of idiot children away from the asylum. The offer was, however, eventually rejected by the County Council Board who was unwilling to finance the additional expense.[34] Despite the lack of success the willingness to extend the grant highlights the eagerness of the LAB in preventing the admission of child patients to asylums. Overcrowding caused in part by the admission of the chronic and harmless was a constant pressure on asylums in Lancashire. At the end of the period in question, the Commissioners in Lunacy conducted their annual inspection of Prestwich Asylum and noted that 'many of the patients we saw appeared to be of the mild class of dements who could be satisfactorily dealt with in workhouses'.[35] Therefore we can see that the problem was one that persisted beyond the chronological parameters of this book.

It must also be recognised that the relationships between urban asylums and their surrounding Poor Law unions, over how to manage the mentally disabled, were not always as cordial as the one experienced between the Prestwich Asylum and the Rochdale Union. The West Derby Poor Law Union in its efforts to move on the pauper insane provided a constant source of friction for the LAB and by extension the asylums of the county. Located in a densely populated part of the city of Liverpool, this union dealt with a large number of lunatics and it was regularly frustrated by its inability to transfer patients to Lancashire's asylums. Links between the Prestwich Asylum and West Derby were tangential, but the role of the LAB in orchestrating provision for Lunacy across Lancashire brought these two institutions closer together. The Guardians of West Derby were particularly averse to accumulating large numbers of chronic and harmless children in their Workhouse. In February 1895 it was recorded that:

> A deputation from the Guardians of the West Derby Union, supported by members of most of the Unions in the County, attended before the Board with reference to the provision of special accommodation for young persons and children of weak intellect.[36]

The West Derby Union was at the forefront of campaigning for extra provision for children with mental illness and disability in Lancashire. Such enthusiasm was not out of concern for the young people of Liverpool, but rather because it did not see its role in the economy of care as having to deal with 'children of weak intellect'. The relationship between the union and the Board was one of tension. As we have seen earlier, it resorted to extreme measures to try and force the LAB to admit more children to the county's asylums. In a letter dated 7 August 1895, the Clerk of the union announced: 'I am directed by the Guardians to inform you that, owing to the overcrowded state of the Mill Road Infirmary, they will be unable to admit any more lunatics for the present'.[37]

These actions had consequences within the city that extended beyond the closed workhouse. The decision to refuse new admissions of pauper lunatics forced a response from the Liverpool Constabulary who were apprehensive about the wider effects of not being able to dispose of lunatics in the workhouse. They were forced to respond and sent their own letter to the LAB, two days later, articulating their concerns:

> As you are aware, Sect. 15 of the Lunacy Act directs constables as well as relieving officers to apprehend wandering lunatics. *In practice* nearly all are apprehended by constables. In Liverpool it has been the universal custom—a custom still holding good in all the Unions, save that of West derby—to receive all lunatics apprehended by the police at the Workhouse Infirmaries… Under the decision of the West Derby Guardians, it will become necessary that lunatics apprehended within the district of the Union be locked up in police cells (most unfit and improper places for the detention of such cases), and looked after for hours, or possibly days, by persons with no experience and no capacity for such duty.[38]

Although the actions of the West Derby Union were drastic, they had a limited impact. The Guardians conceded that closing the infirmary to new admissions only caused a rush of new acute cases when the closure was removed.[39] These efforts, on the part of the Poor Law Union, display the tensions that having to maintain and fund pauper insanity could have on local welfare provision. Despite their failure, the union continued to use closure as a threat when their infirmary became overcrowded and they could not transfer patients to asylums. While the LAB searched for a solution to the problem of the ever-growing number of lunatics, including the extension of the 4*s.* grant already mentioned, the West Derby Union relentlessly continued its pressure campaign. In December 1895 the Union School was inspected by the Inspector of Poor Law Schools who reported:

> There are a few weak-minded children whose cases the Guardians might specially consider—Phoebe Dorey (8), who should, if possible, be sent to an institution for imbecile children, also Elizabeth Cowie (8), Douglas Davies (15), and Alfred Rawsthorne (14), who might possibly so be sent.[40]

By using the School's Inspector the Guardians sought to reinforce and legitimise its need for alternative provision for these children. Their concerns were eventually eased when the LAB agreed that the new Lancashire asylum, being built at Winwick Hall, would be used to accommodate some chronic and harmless child cases. The proviso for this arrangement was that cases could only be transferred from other asylums and there were to be no new cases direct from Poor Law unions. The intention was to free space in existing asylums for acute cases. The new Winwick Asylum would, however, take four years to build and did not offer any instant amelioration of the overcrowding problems. To solve the issue with more immediacy the West Derby Union called on more external support and complained directly to the Commissioners in Lunacy in London. The Commissioners sided with the Union and decreed, in a letter to the LAB, that:

> The matter is one of such grave public importance that, though reluctant to do so, the Commissioners would suggest, for the consideration of the Lancashire Asylums Board, the erection of temporary accommodation at one or other of the Lancashire Asylums, pending the completion of the Asylum at Winwick.[41]

The continued actions of West Derby Guardians, and the interjection of the Commissioners in Lunacy, forced the LAB to seek a more rapid solution to the issue of overcrowding and ease the strain that large numbers of chronic and harmless placed on space inside Lancashire's asylums. Consequently, a committee was established to try and find adequate alternative provision for the chronic and harmless that led to the arrangement with the Derby Asylum at Mickleover mentioned above.[42] It is evident that the mixed economy of care at times caused friction as well as cooperation. In this instance Poor Law Guardians were able to circumvent the admission procedures of asylums and force them to take more patients. These circumstances reinforce the limited role that the asylum had in selecting its own patients and demonstrate that child mental health was an important welfare issue that extended beyond the specialised sphere of the asylum.

In early 1895, before the spat with West Derby, the LAB received another resolution, this time from the Poor Law Union at Ulverston in the north of the county. This correspondence indicates that the issue of chronic and harmless children was a tension felt all over and was not just a problem of the large urban centres such as Manchester and Liverpool. The resolution from Ulverston noted:

> These persons [imbeciles], whilst classed as lunatics by the Law, are not really persons who should be confined in the ordinary Lunatic Asylums … especially in the present over-crowded condition of the Asylums. The present practice of confining them … with sane persons in workhouses, is most undesirable … especially in the case of children of weak intellect associating with those who are not so afflicted. That it is the opinion of this Board that separate institutions should be provided for the treatment of the above, where they may be beneficially occupied … and receive training suitable to their special condition. That the cost of dealing with this class of persons ought not to fall exclusively on the Poor Rate, but should be provided for out of Imperial Taxation.[43]

The Ulverston correspondence is important for a number of reasons. First of all it acknowledged that Poor Law Guardians were aware and supportive of the asylum's stance that harmless and chronic patients should not be confined within the institutions. Secondly, it also demonstrated the widespread lack of enthusiasm for confining these patients with the able-bodied in workhouses. Finally, the Ulverston correspondence displays unwillingness on the part of Poor Law Guardians to be responsible for the cost of chronic and harmless patients, either in the asylum or workhouse, and shows that they felt central government should make a contribution towards their care. A similar stance was adopted by the Chorlton Guardians who argued that 'the whole cost of maintaining lunatics and imbecile persons … should be borne by the nation at large'.[44] Consequently, the issue of child mental disability was considered an 'Imperial' issue and it was argued that it should have been financed accordingly.

The spectrum of attitudes within the mixed economy of care that related to mentally impaired children were not just evident in Manchester. The asylums of Birmingham and Colney Hatch provide further evidence of extensive networks for managing insane children. In Birmingham the workhouse infirmary was a key space for dealing with children, some of which were eventually transferred to the asylum. In the summer of 1882 the workhouse increased its capacity to deal with children in its own infirmary, rather than moving them to the asylum. New male and female nurses for the epileptic wards were employed, with such investment demonstrating an effort to keep epileptic children outside of the asylum.[45] Previously the Birmingham Union had transferred this type of patient directly to the county institution. The last of which was William Stanley, an epileptic who at the age of 9 was admitted to the asylum from the workhouse in 1881.[46]

Much like in asylums, the Birmingham Workhouse used inmates to help run the institution. One of the older children, Rebecca Bennett, 'an imbecile who is classed as able bodied' was employed as a night nurse for the whole of 1884 in the Female Bedridden Ward.[47] Children were thus coerced into being useful in workhouses regardless of their mental health conditions. But much like the experience in Manchester, the relationship between mental health and the Poor Law was not always an easy one. Dr Suckling, the Birmingham Poor Law Union Workhouse physician complained, in 1884, about the number of insane patients in the infirmary. At a meeting with the Guardians he stated 'that Medical Officers outside constantly send persons of unsound mind to the Workhouse instead of sending them straight to the asylum'.[48] In this instance the medical staff saw the asylum as the preferred option for the insane, and it again emphasised the inability of the institutions to select their own patients.[49] Dr Suckling's background is not documented, but he was keen to move on all patients that suffered from mental illness or disability.

For children suffering from learning disabilities in Birmingham the Borough Asylum at Winson Green became a less likely destination for them as the period progressed. The Rubery Hill Asylum was, however, more often utilised both by the asylum for transferring patients and by the Poor Law Union for sending new admissions. In 1884 the sub-committee responsible for the infirmary at the Birmingham Workhouse declared, 'the most desirable way to remove the pressure in the sick wards of the workhouse would be by the removal of some of the cases of epileptics and imbeciles of both sexes to Rubery Hill Lunatic Asylum thus making portions of those wards available for the treatment of ordinary sick cases'.[50] Rubery Hill was a pressure valve that eased overcrowding in the asylum and the sick wards of the Union that was caused by long stay patients such as epileptics and imbeciles.

There is also evidence that the asylum was thought of, and accessed, as a general medical institution. In 1903 'the Medical Officer reported that Catherine Morley, Probationer Nurse, had been removed to the Borough Asylum, suffering with scarlett fever'.[51] Morley was not a child, but she also was not certified as insane. Removing such cases shows that the asylum fulfilled a number of medical roles.[52] The Superintendent of Devon County Asylum and prominent alienist, John C. Bucknill, was frustrated by Poor Law Medical Officers 'whom he believed sent dying people to him knowing he would admit them and therefore nurse them up to their death in his institution'.[53] The asylum therefore was not always eager to fulfil the multiple roles that it was given by external institutions, although it had little choice in avoiding them.

Much like in Manchester, a broader landscape of care can also be observed in Birmingham. The Poor Law Unions of the city did not just rely on the nearby borough asylum to dispose of its harmless and chronic patients but used a number of smaller private establishments also. One of these was located at Edgbaston Grove. The records for this smaller institution no longer exist but some of its correspondence with the Birmingham Union Poor Law Guardians has survived. In 1888 the problem of overcrowding was evident and given voice by the private asylum's superintendent G.B. Lloyd:

> I … urge your colleagues at the Board of Guardians to give way to the extent of being willing to take back the 45 to 50 harmless imbeciles who are still fit to be removed to a workhouse, and to retain future cases of a similar kind; as I doubt if it was ever intended for that the lunacy law should be used for such persons.
>
> The case of the outborough Aston patients placed with us, instead of at Hatton, (or at greater distances under contract) must be carefully reconsidered also by us.
>
> I had been under the impression that we were doing good in receiving them, so long as we were paid enough to cover interest and maintenance but the feeling yesterday seemed to press in the opposite direction.[54]

It is apparent that a significant number of harmless patients had been deposited at Edgbaston Grove which the institution wanted to return to the Birmingham Union, primarily it seems, because it was no longer economically viable to keep them. The question was also raised about the use of the lunacy laws and whether these were suitable patients to be confined. Such a statement is interesting because the Idiots Act, introduced in 1886, had sought to define the differences between 'lunatics', 'idiots' and 'imbeciles'. It might be that such distinctions permeated this situation. Despite the eagerness of Edgbaston Grove to return the patients, the Birmingham Guardians were not so keen and responded 'that at the present time the Epileptic wards are overcrowded and that when the new infirmary is opened there will be no extra accommodation for them so that it will be impossible to take any cases back from the asylum'.[55] Just as in Manchester, responsibility for the chronic and harmless was a source of tension. The surviving records unfortunately do not provide any detail of how this disagreement was resolved, but there is no evidence that the imbecile patients at Edgbaston Grove were returned to the workhouse or deposited in the asylum.

Special education was also a development of this period. From 1898, the Committee for Special Schools in Birmingham sought to divert children from the asylum and towards educational provision. This was a clear shift from what had gone before and saw non-medically trained teachers used to identify children that were considered to be unable to deal with the intellectual rigours of mainstream schooling. The effectiveness of this method can be assessed by looking at the admissions data for Birmingham in Fig. 4.1 (above) where the rate of admission peaks before 1898. The Committee had a number of key duties. It decided 'what children shall be sent to classes for Blind, Deaf and Defective Children'. It moreover made recommendations on the nature of teaching and the teachers to be appointed, as well as the prosecution of parents whose children were not attending school regularly. They likewise decided when children needed to be sent to other institutions, which children should be removed, and 'to take the general superintendence of all matters connected with the interests of the Blind, Deaf and Feeble-minded Children'.[56]

The emergence of educational establishments for the mentally disabled proved to be popular in Birmingham. The school for feeble-minded children was filled to capacity by 14 March 1899 and the committee was already looking for further space to provide for the city's mentally impaired youth.[57] Such popularity meant that the committee needed to be selective in the children that it sent to these schools. Regardless of the measures introduced to manage children with mental illnesses and disabilities they were often unable to keep up with the demand that they placed on provision. By 1903 there were forty-one children with learning disabilities aged under thirteen that attended the Birmingham School Board's special classes, in the same year only one child was admitted to the borough asylum at Winson Green.[58] The success of Birmingham's schools was not replicated countrywide and it is crucial to continue to focus on the differences that occurred between regions.

Variations in Use

To date, the importance of the locality in relation to the operation and management of county asylums has been examined in three ways. Firstly, asylums have been located in a vertical system of governance and their relationships with government legislation and the Commissioners in Lunacy have been assessed.[59] There is often a focus on the dominance of the centre over the periphery and the implementation of regulations in this approach.[60] The second view has had a horizontal focus and has highlighted the importance of the asylum in a local landscape of institutional provision for the insane.[61] Both outlooks have implied that asylums operated in a standardised way, with variations in their attitude towards the control of government and the authority of the Commissioners. The method adopted in this book has been deliberately horizontal, looking at how the asylums related to the institutions of the localities in which they operated, but also the power structures installed by central government and the debates about their effectiveness have been acknowledged.

Thirdly, the literature has placed the asylum in its Poor Law context.[62] This has improved understanding of how welfare networks operated and has shown how the Poor Law and insane institutions worked together. Greater insight into the individual influence of Guardians, the patients to be transferred, and medical ideas of insanity have all been revealed with this approach. Scholars have, however, overlooked a number of key things that have been highlighted here. Specific patient populations and their experiences have been ignored. The arguments have largely been a top-down assessment of the Poor Law systems, and the role of the asylum within a broad network of provision has not been assessed until now. Most importantly, it has always been assumed that pauper institutions operated as part of a wider system but institutional comparisons have been nevertheless neglected.

With regards to the Poor Law we know that relief was not standardised and there was no centralised mechanism for dealing with poverty, especially amongst vulnerable groups such as children.[63] Rather, responses and sentiments towards welfare, relief, and the poor were defined at local levels.[64] How the county asylum system was affected by such a varied application of the Poor Law has not been fully developed. Attempts to do so have addressed the issue broadly and have not considered specific patient populations. There are two substantial historiographical case studies that present differing outlooks towards the county pauper asylum from the Poor Law. These are located in Devon and Northamptonshire (in the period before the opening of Berrywood in 1876). In Devon, pressure from local elites forced the building of a county asylum before the legislation of 1845 had passed, while the Northamptonshire elites resisted pressure to build a county institution until 1876.[65] Both examples emphasise the importance of local concerns and apathy towards government interference.

Of the five asylums examined, Northamptonshire as a county is the most accessible for the purposes here. The experience of Lancashire is complicated by the four large asylums of the county and the incomplete nature of Poor Law records from the Manchester area; Birmingham was a borough asylum that only served three heavily urbanised unions; the Three Counties Asylum had a catchment area that spanned across three separate counties and numerous Poor Law Unions; and Colney Hatch's proximity to the capital makes it difficult to succinctly gain access to the attitudes of the various influences impacting on admissions. Northamptonshire was made up of a manageable twelve Poor Law Unions. They were diverse in nature but all accessed the county asylum located at Berrywood after 1876. At this time the county stretched from Peterborough in the east to Towcester in the south-west, meaning it spanned much of rural central England. Its location therefore makes it an important historical prism to gauge a number of attitudes.

The boundaries of Poor Law Unions in Northamptonshire were drawn to reinforce the significant influence of the local landed gentry.[66] The Brackley Poor Law Union was dominated by the Cartwright family; Sir Charles Knightley was resident in Daventry; Edward Bouverie and the Marquess of Northampton in Hardingstone; the Fermors in Towcester; Lords Cardigan, Wesmoreland, Montagu and Winchelsea at Oundle; Earl Fitzwilliam and the Marquees of Exeter at Peterborough; and Earl Spencer at Brixworth.[67] The Poor Law Union map appeased these influences and left the Northampton Union itself as 'one of the few poor law boardrooms in the country where middle-class professionals, tradesmen and a shopkeeping elite had some influence'.[68] Cathy Smith argues that those advocating for a county asylum in Northamptonshire were the local gentry and well-to-do that dominated the rural unions.[69] Despite such influential support there were still disparate approaches and attitudes towards the asylum once it was built. These difference are revealed, and to an extent masked, by the admissions of children from around the county of Northamptonshire to the asylum after 1876.

Table 4.3 reveals the varied use of the Northamptonshire asylum. The unions containing the county's large towns (Northampton, Wellingborough, and Kettering) were the most frequent users of asylum provision as one would expect. In the remaining, mostly rural unions, there appears to have been a uniform approach to sending children to the asylum. Such an assumption is, however, misleading and the data masks a variety of attitudes towards poverty and the asylum. From the table it might be expected that the Daventry Union was hostile towards the asylum, only sending three children during the period. A more accurate description would be that Daventry was ambivalent towards the asylum. The Union Workhouse had a lunatic ward where it confined some of its insane and the Guardians were not averse to awarding out-relief payments to prevent cases, either child or adult, being admitted to the workhouse

Table 4.3 Admissions to the Northamptonshire Asylum by local Poor Law Unions

Poor Law Union	*Male*	*Female*	*Total*
Brackley	8	1	9
Brixworth	3	2	5
Daventry	0	3	3
Hardingstone	6	0	6
Kettering	13	13	26
Northampton	22	20	42
Oundle	1	3	4
Peterborough	4	3	7
Potterspury	8	2	10
Thrapston	5	3	8
Towcester	1	4	5
Wellingborough	15	13	28

Source: NRO, Male Patient Casebooks, NCLA/6/2/2/1-12; NRO Female Patient Casebooks, NCLA/6/2/1/1-13

or the asylum.[70] This was very much in contrast to the Brixworth Union a prominent crusading union that sought to eradicate expenditure on the sick poor.[71] All of the children admitted from Brixworth were sent to the asylum from the lunatic ward of the Workhouse. This suggests that an initial period of assessment took place before the Guardians were satisfied that the expense of asylum confinement was necessary.[72] On the other hand, Peterborough, a reasonably sized cathedral town and located at the periphery of the county, only admitted seven children to the asylum and instead preferred to focus on providing out-relief to families in need.[73]

It has often been assumed that cost was a factor for retaining or disposing of the pauper insane.[74] Workhouses were thought to provide a less expensive alternative to asylum care. But it can be seen that cost was not a major issue and a range of local concerns, such as heightened enthusiasm for providing outdoor relief, impacted on attitudes towards the asylum and shaped admissions to them. Also, the introduction of the 4*s*. grant did not lead to a rush in certifications as expected.[75] The admission of children to the Northamptonshire asylum from outside of the county further suggests that cost was not a factor and that counties were willing to pay a premium in order to accommodate their pauper insane.

Conclusion

It is evident that there were varied systems of care in operation for the pauper insane child during the period. A number of important findings have been uncovered. Firstly, the position of children in a broader context of managing and disposing of the insane has been demonstrated. Previously, adult patients had been the sole focus, but now the experience and movement of children through the multiple spaces of welfare has been explored. We can see that children were an important element in a wider economy of care that has hitherto largely been neglected. The role that they occupied is essential to the historiography of asylums because they were the incurable and harmless patients that Scull suggested clogged up the system and damaged the curative reputation of the institution.[76] Often the asylum was not the first resort for these patients. Children were part of a mixed landscape of medical provision dealing with insanity and their participation did not just contribute to overcrowding in asylums, but also impacted on the management and organisation of workhouses and private institutions. The movement of children through the care network may best be described as a series of campaigns, complaints, and congestion.

It has also been revealed that established towns and cities were better equipped to deal with insane children in the mid to late nineteenth century. They managed to develop a range of responses to child mental disability and illness that will feature in the next chapter. The literature had assumed that access to alternative provisions had only been a feature in London and had not been developed in the provinces during the nineteenth century.[77] A range of extra provision for the insane outside of the capital demonstrates that there was an assortment of relief methods, and these findings help to better understand the treatment of the insane in both urban and rural areas.

Moreover, the discovery of a wider network of provision than previously acknowledged, has led to a revision of the role of the asylum. It has long been acknowledged that the idea of asylums as Foucauldian institutions of confinement and control is simplistic and problematic. Through an examination of the destinations where children were admitted from, and subsequently dispatched to, a layer of nuance has been added to the argument here. Asylums were not solely magnets for the unwanted, but fluid systems that accommodated a range of patients and numerous conditions. The differing roles and functions that they served were often dependent upon geographic location and the prevailing attitudes of influential gentleman outside of the institution. Such conclusions further reinforce the argument that there was not a coherent or unified system of asylum provision in England during the second half of the nineteenth century.

Such diversity in the asylum network is emphasised by experiences in Northamptonshire. The Berrywood Asylum that served the county was viewed in different ways by its local Poor Law Unions. By situating patients at the centre of the analysis it is possible to adopt a lens that examines the relationship between Poor Law and asylum. A number of problems and shortcomings are raised, however. There is an opportunity for the scope of this argument to be extended. It might be asked how the same methods could be adopted to better understand the treatment of other patient populations such as the elderly, women, or illness defined groups. There is also a springboard to build in other regional studies to develop a broader picture of how the insane were managed. While the conclusions provide a new angle for looking at the mixed economy of medical provision, a more in-depth study of regionality has the potential to develop a better understanding of the fractured nature of care for the insane in the second half of the nineteenth century.

Perhaps the most important question raised from the chapter is: what happened to children that did not find their way to asylums, or were removed from the mixed economy of care offered by the Poor Law/asylum systems? The response to such a question is complex and moves beyond the asylum towards a range of alternative provision, both state and privately funded, that we must now explore.

Notes

1. L. Smith, 'The County Asylum in the Mixed Economy of Care, 1808–1845,' in J. Melling and B. Forsythe (eds.), *Insanity, Institutions, and Society, 1800–1914: A Social History of Madness in Comparative Perspective* (London: Routledge, 1999), pp. 33–47.
2. C. Smith, 'Parsimony, Power, and Prescriptive Legislation: The Politics of Pauper Lunacy in Northamptonshire, 1845–1876,' *Bulletin of the History of Medicine*, 81/2 (2007), pp. 359–385, p. 366; P. Bartlett and D. Wright (eds.), *Outside the Walls of the Asylum: The History of Care in the Community* (London: Athone, 1999).
3. L. Smith, '"A Sad Spectacle of Hopeless Mental Degradation": The Management of the Insane in West Midlands Workhouses, 1815–60,' in J. Reinarz and L. Schwarz (eds.), *Medicine and the Workhouse* (Woodbridge: Boydell & Brewer, 2013), pp. 103–122; P. Bartlett, *The Poor Law of Lunacy: The Administration of Pauper Lunatics in Mid-Nineteenth-Century England* (London: University of Leicester Press, 1999); P. Bartlett, 'The Asylum and the Poor Law: The Productive Alliance,' in J. Melling and B. Forsythe (eds.), *Insanity, Institutions and Society*, pp. 48–67; P. Bartlett, 'The Asylum, the Workhouse, and the Voice of the Insane Poor in Nineteenth-Century-England,' *International Journal of Law and Psychiatry*, 24/4 (1998), pp. 421–432; J.K. Walton, 'Casting Out and Bringing Back in Victorian England: Pauper Lunatics 1840–1870,' *The Anatomy of Madness*, vol. 2, pp. 132–146; C. Smith, 'Family, Community and the Victorian Asylum: A Case Study of Northampton General Lunatic Asylum and its Pauper Lunatics,' *Family and Community History*, 9/2 (2006), pp. 109–124, suggested that asylums were used strategically by families at times. Mark Finnane, 'Asylums, Families and the State,' *History Workshop Journal*, 20 (1985), pp. 134–148.
4. A. Scull, *Museums of Madness: Madness and Society in Britain 1700–1900* (London: Allen Lane, 1979); Scull, *The Most Solitary of Afflictions: Madness and Society in Britain 1700–1900* (London: Yale University Press, 1993); D. Mellet, *The Prerogative of Asylumdom: Social, Cultural and Administrative Aspects of the Institutional Treatment of the Insane in*

Nineteenth Century Britain (London: Garland, 1982); C. Smith, 'Family, Community and the Victorian Asylum'; C. Smith, "Living with Insanity: Narratives of Poverty, Pauperism and Sickness in Asylum records 1840–76,' in A. Gestrich, E. Hurren, and S. King (eds.), *Poverty and Sickness in Modern Europe: Narratives of the Sick Poor, 1780–1938* (London: Continuum, 2012), pp. 117–142.

5. BCA, All Saints Asylum, Male Casebook 4, MS344/12/4, George Clift, p. 62.
6. LMA, Friern Hospital (Colney Hatch), Female Casebook 3, H12/CH/B/11/003a, Susan Squires.
7. LMA, Friern Hospital (Colney Hatch), Male Casebook 33, H12/CH/B/13/033, John Feltham, p. 140.
8. LMA, Friern Hospital (Colney Hatch), Male Casebook 49, H12/CH/B/13/049, Thomas Walker, p. 134.
9. For example some northern industrial poor law unions had lunatic wards that could hold over 100 patients, see F. Driver, *Power and Pauperism: The Workhouse System, 1834–1884* (Cambridge: Cambridge University Press, 1993), pp. 160–161.
10. LMA, Friern Hospital (Colney Hatch), Male Casebook 18, H12/CH/B/13/018, Alfred Morran, Admission no. 4952.
11. LMA, Friern Hospital (Colney Hatch), Male Casebook 44, H12/CH/B/13/044, Alfred Sowter, Admission no. 12634.
12. BCA, All Saints Asylum, Female Casebook, MS344/12/42, Maria Butler, p. 62.
13. LRO, Prestwich, Male Casebook 1, QAM6/6/1, Edward Ridings, Admission no. 68.
14. BLA, Three Counties, Male Casebook 2, LF31/2, John Beale, Admission no. 1292, p. 1.
15. BLA, Three Counties, Male Casebook 2, LF31/2, Edwin Seabrook, Admission no. 1380, pp. 43–45; BLA, Three Counties, Male Casebook 2, LF31/2, John Prutton, Admission no. 1554, p. 120; BLA, Three Counties, Male Casebook 2, LF31/2, Alfred Lester, Admission no. 1654, p. 168; BLA, Three Counties, Male Casebook 3, LF31/3, Henry Aylett, Admission no. 2384, p. 125 and p. 319; BLA, Three Counties, Female Casebook 12, LF29/12, Ada Harding, Admission no. 6577, p. 39.
16. NRO, St Crispin Collection, Male Casebook 3, NCLA/6/2/2/3, Charles York, Admission no. 1196, pp. 147–149; NRO, St Crispin Collection, Male Casebook 4, NCLA/6/2/2/4, Joseph Harris, Admission no. 1550, p. 39; NRO, St Crispin Collection, Female Casebook 5, NCLA/6/2/1/, Lucy Jones, Admission no. 2242, p. 175; NRO, St Crispin Collection, Female Casebook 6, NCLA/6/2/1/6, Elizabeth Robinson, Admission no. 2696, p. 74.

17. BLA, Three Counties, Female Casebook 2, LF29/2, Priscilla Elliot, Admission no. 1413, p. 60.
18. D. Wright, 'Learning Disability and the New Poor Law in England, 1834–1867,' *Disability and Society*, 15/5 (2000), pp. 731–745, p. 741.
19. A. Tomkins, 'Paupers and the Infirmary in Mid-Eighteenth-Century Shrewsbury,' *Medical History*, 43/2 (1999), pp. 208–227.
20. LRO, Prestwich, Male Casebook 33, QAM6/6/33, Joseph Smith, Admission no. 7655.
21. BCA, All Saints Asylum, Male Casebook 5, MS344/12/5, William Binton, p. 78.
22. LRO, Prestwich, Male Casebook 18, QAM6/6/18, Frederick Bowcock, Admission no. 4394.
23. LMA, Friern Hospital (Colney Hatch), Male Casebook 1, H12/CH/B/13/001, James Gray, Admission no. 426.
24. LMA, Friern Hospital (Colney Hatch), Female Casebook 1a, H12/CH/B/11/001a, Mary Ann Beard, Admission no. 876.
25. Bartlett, 'The Productive Alliance'; Bartlett, *The Poor Law of Lunacy*; Forsythe, Melling, and Adair, 'The New Poor Law and the County Pauper Lunatic Asylum—The Devon Experience 1834–1884,' *Social History of Medicine*, 9/3 (1996), pp. 335–355; Wright, 'Learning Disability'; Adair, Forsythe, and Melling, 'A Danger to the Public? Disposing of Pauper Lunatics in Late Victorian and Edwardian England: Plympton St. Mary Union and the Devon County Asylum, 1867–1914,' *Medical History*, 42/1 (1998), pp. 1–25.
26. Wright, *Mental Disability in Victorian England: The Earlswood Asylum, 1847–1901* (Oxford: Clarendon, 2001), p. 17.
27. GMCRO, Proceedings of the Lancashire Asylums Board and Arrival Reports of County Asylums, A/Pres/Box 647 1894–1912.
28. Lancashire Asylums Board, A/Pres/Box 647 1894–1912.
29. GMCRO, Lancashire Asylums Board, A/Pres/Box 647, p. 67.
30. NRO, St Crispin Collection, Accounts Book, NCLA/2/18/2/1, Out of Counties 1 pp. 820–828.
31. GMCRO, Proceedings of the Lancashire Asylums Board, A/Pres/Box 647, 28 November 1895, p. 16.
32. K. Jones, *A History of the Mental Health Services* (London: Routledge and Kegan Paul, 1972), p. 161; Scull, *Most Solitary*, p. 308.
33. L. Ray, 'Models of Madness in Victorian Asylum Practice,' *European Journal of Sociology*, 22 (1981), pp. 229–264, pp. 252–253; Rob Ellis, 'Reassessment of the Four-Shilling Grant'.
34. Report of the Commissioners in Lunacy, 1907, included in the proceedings of Lancashire Asylums Board, A/Pres/Box647, 1907.
35. Proceedings of the Lancashire Asylums Board, A/Pres/Box647, 1907.

36. Proceedings of the Lancashire Asylums Board, A/Pres/Box 647, 28 February 1895, p. 5.
37. Ibid., pp. 5–6.
38. Ibid., 29 August 1895, p. 6.
39. Ibid., 19 July 1898, p. 61.
40. Ibid., 28 November 1896, p. 8.
41. Ibid., 26 August 1897, p. 63.
42. Ibid., 1895, 29 August 1895, p. 7.
43. Ibid., 1895, p. 6.
44. *The Manchester Guardian*, 'Chorlton Board of Guardians,' 29 February 1868, p. 5.
45. BCA, Birmingham Union Infirmary Sub-Committee, GP/B/2/4/1/1, 28 July 1882.
46. BCA, All Saints Asylum, Index male 12/4, William Stanley, Admission no. 5219.
47. BCA, Infirmary Sub-Committee, GP/B/2/4/1/1, 27 October 1882.
48. BCA, Infirmary Sub-Committee, GP/B/2/4/1/2, 4 il 1884.
49. J. Walton, 'Lunacy in the Industrial Revolution: A Study of Asylum Admissions in Lancashire, 1848–1850,' *Journal of Social History*, 13/1 (1979–1980), pp. 1–22, p. 4.
50. BCA, Infirmary Sub-Committee, GP/B/2/4/1/2, 28 November 1884.
51. BCA, Infirmary Sub-Committee, GP/B/2/4/1/2, 20 January 1903.
52. C. Smith, 'Living with Insanity'.
53. Melling et al., 'The New Poor Law,' p. 340.
54. BCA, Infirmary Sub-Committee, GP/B/2/4/1/4, 6 June 1888.
55. Ibid.
56. BCA, Birmingham Education Committee Special Schools Committee of the School Board Minutes 10 February 1898–17 March 1903, SB/B11/1/1/1, 10 February 1898, pp. 1–2.
57. Ibid., 14 March 1899, p. 46.
58. Ibid.
59. E.D. Myers, 'Workhouse or Asylum: The Nineteenth Century Battle for the Care of the Pauper Insane,' *Psychiatric Bulletin*, 22/9 (1998), pp. 575–577; C. Smith, 'Parsimony, Power, and Prescriptive Legislation'; N. Hervey, 'A Slavish Bowing Down: The Lunacy Commission and the Psychiatric Profession,' in Bynum et al., *Anatomy of Madness*, vol. 2, pp. 98–131.
60. A. Scull, *Most Solitary of Afflictions*; R. Porter, *Mind Forg'd Manacles: A History of Madness in England from the Restoration to Regency* (London: Athlone, 1987), p. 287.
61. B. Forsythe, J. Melling, and R. Adair, 'Politics of Lunacy: Central State Regulation and the Devon Pauper Lunatic Asylum, 1845–1914,' in Melling and Forsythe (eds.), *Insanity, Institutions*; Pamela Michael, *Care*

and Treatment of the Mentally Ill in North Wales, 1800–2000 (Cardiff: University of Wales Press, 2003); A. Digby, *Madness, Morality and Medicine: A Study of the York Retreat, 1796–1914* (Cambridge: Cambridge University Press, 1985); R. Hunter and I. MacAlpine, *Psychiatry for the Poor:1851 Colney Hatch Asylum—Friern Hospital 1973: A Medical and Social History* (London: Dawsons 1974); Bartlett and Wright (eds.), *Outside the Walls of the Asylum*; P. Bartlett, 'The Productive Alliance'.

62. Melling et al., 'The New Poor Law'; Bartlett, *Poor Law of Lunacy*; A. Suzuki, 'The Politics and Ideology of Non-Restraint: The Case of Hanwell Asylum,' *Medical History*, 39/1 (1995), pp. 1–17; Wright 'Learning Disability'; E. Miller, 'Variations in the Official Prevalence and Disposal of the Insane in England under the Poor Law, 1850–1900,' *History of Psychiatry*, 18/1 (2007), pp. 25–38.
63. S. King, *Poverty and Welfare in England 1700–1850* (Manchester: Manchester University Press, 2000).
64. Ibid.
65. Melling, 'New Poor Law'; C. Smith, 'Parsimony, Power and Prescriptive Legislation'.
66. Hurren, *Protesting About Pauperism: Poverty, Politics and Poor Relief in Late-Victorian England, 1870–1900* (London: Boydell & Brewer, 2008), p. 82.
67. Ibid., pp. 82–84.
68. Ibid., p. 83.
69. Cathy Smith, 'Parsimony, Power, and Prescriptive Legislation,' p. 361.
70. NRO, Daventry Lunatic Register, PL3/306, 1896–1901; Daventry Guardians Minutes, PL3/13-19, 1874–1894.
71. Hurren, *Protesting*.
72. NRO, Brixworth Union, Register of Lunatics, PL2/203
73. NRO, Peterborough Guardian Minutes, PL8/19-23, 1874–1889.
74. Ellis, 'Reassessment of the 4*s*. Grant'.
75. Miller, 'Variations in the Official Prevalence and Disposal of the Insane,' p. 32; Ellis ibid.
76. Scull, *Museums*; *The Most Solitary of Afflictions*.
77. Wright, 'Learning Disability and the Poor Law'.

CHAPTER 5

Beyond the Asylum: Dealing with Insane Children

It can now be observed that child mental ill-health and disability was managed across an economy of care largely operated by local officials and institutions under the jurisdiction of state legislation. The Poor Law played a dominant role in responding to the needs of the sick poor and subsequently offered numerous avenues of care, such as the workhouse, infirmary, or asylum. It was not, however, the only welfare option available to the pauper insane. By further widening our focus it is possible to explore the methods of managing mentally impaired children that extended beyond the medical provisions of the publicly funded Poor Law. Attention turns to the development of schooling and education, the emergence of hospitals for children, philanthropic efforts that ranged from confinement to migration, and domestic care. It is notable that many of the spaces to be discussed have received relatively sparse attention from historians of psychiatry. The domestic environment has featured in the recent historiography, but the remainder have been conspicuously overlooked.[1] By reassessing the care options for children the chapter traces a trend of increased intervention in the lives of children from individuals, the state, and philanthropy.

Education

With regards to child development, the introduction of elementary education was the most important legislation introduced during the nineteenth century. It is essential to establish at the outset how elementary

S.J. Taylor, *Child Insanity in England, 1845-1907*, Palgrave Studies in the History of Childhood, DOI 10.1007/978-1-137-60027-1_5

schooling in Britain from 1870 played a pivotal role in the identification and management of the mentally inferior child. The numerous Education Acts between 1870 and 1891 created an education system that was both compulsory and free for those aged up to ten years old, and thus thrust the intellectual abilities of children into a wider arena than had been experienced by any generation previously. That does not, however, mean that education was without social significance in the years preceding the first Elementary Education Act, or as it is more commonly known 'Forster's Act' of 1870. Before the legislation there were already two million children registered in schools across the country, a figure equivalent to 13 % of the population, and Sunday Schools provided educational provision for a further 525,000.[2] While this figure might seem impressive, education was often interrupted by a need for children to contribute to the family economy or in order to fulfil domestic duties while their parents were working.[3] Nevertheless, families were aware of the value attached to obtaining an education and scholarship has observed that families used schooling to build the human capital of their children and to interact with written rules and popular culture in the years before 1870.[4] Furthermore, in many rural areas families prioritised the education of able-bodied children and had to calculate which of their offspring should be educated first. Such actions allowed the possibility of better employment, perhaps in the burgeoning railway industry, and consequently increased contributions to the family economy. Within these discussions of education, and its benefits, those that were unable to improve through schooling have been neglected.

Alongside the principle of universal education, Forster's Education Act also established local school boards that were responsible not only for the building and maintenance of schools but also the attendance of youngsters to populate them. Inevitably, such a change was not without its challenges and Eric Hopkins identifies that perhaps the biggest 'was to teach the residuum who had not previously attended school'.[5] A class divide emerged where parents who could afford to pay the fee for church schools continued to do so, while those that could not sent their children to be educated with the local school board. Parents who were aware that their offspring were 'slow' or incapable of learning consequently dispatched them to congregate in the classes of the local school board because they were not worth the investment of a fee-paying education. In such a permissive environment it would have been simpler to keep a child with mental impairments at home and away from prying eyes, at least until 1880 when education became compulsory for all children aged up to ten.

The nineteen years between the Elementary Education Act of 1880 and the Elementary Education (Epileptic and Defective Children) Act of 1899 were an educative vacuum for children who lacked the intellectual abilities for conventional learning. The 1880 legislation made attendance at school compulsory, but provision for those with learning difficulties or special education needs was not introduced until the 1899 legislation. Between these years the mentally impaired child was left to get by in tiered mainstream lessons. The expectation was that children would have reached Standard IV by the age of ten; in reality only 47 % of children reached such a level and the lower ability school classes would have been clogged with those unable to reach the national average.[6] This situation was exacerbated by the economic reality of teachers being paid in accordance with their results, thus de-incentivising the education of mentally impaired children. The unsuitability of this situation for the individuals involved is apparent, but the experience is also central to understanding how and why schools played a vital role in identifying the mentally deficient child in the late nineteenth century.

It was inevitable that schools were forced to fulfil a medical role for children of the poor. This did not just cover those that were mentally inadequate but also the malnourished, those in need of dental care, and the visually or hearing impaired.[7] Indeed, the school became the vanguard of identifying medical defects in children and a symbolic intervention by the state in the life and welfare of working-class families.[8] By 1907, and the end of the period under scrutiny, the creation of the School Medical Service saw the responsibility for the identification, classification, and improvement of the child with learning difficulties shift from the medical sphere to an educational one.

The relationship between the spheres of education and medicine was not just about the underperformance of children but it also had a function at a national level. The late nineteenth century was a time when Britain was being challenged on a global scale for the first time and anxiety about losing its international status was linked to fears about national degeneracy that were driven by influential eugenicist ideas. The period saw an increased belief in the need for an educated and healthy working class that was capable of maintaining the empire.[9] With the outbreak of the Boer War in 1899, the educational defects of recruits from the working class became more apparent and fuelled such fears.[10] The elementary school thus became the site to provide moral instruction to the children of the urban poor and in turn help to raise the condition of the most disadvantaged in society.[11] In this social mind-set the only thought given to those with mental impairments was how to prevent such conditions occurring, rather than improvement.

Developing Special Education

Before 1899 provision for those with special educational needs developed slowly and was piecemeal in nature. In addition to the mainstream classes offered by local school boards there were residential schools that provided custodial roles as well as educational. The Darenth School, administered by the Metropolitan Asylums Board (MAB), was one of these institutions. The educational landscape of the late-nineteenth century did not allow for grey areas, which meant that children 'at the elementary schools were treated as normal, those at Darenth and the asylums as imbeciles'.[12] Therefore the mentally incapable that remained in schools were offered an education that they could not access and those at Darenth were denied instruction at a level they could engage with. Such inadequacies were apparent to some and there were campaigns to introduce specialised education. The first of these in 1884 was led by Dr George E. Shuttleworth, the Medical Superintendent of the Royal Albert Idiot Asylum, and Dr Francis Warner, a physician at a number of London's children's hospitals. We can thus see that interest in the educational development of the mentally deficient child was propelled by medical professionals rather than educationalists.

The Darenth School was established in 1878 to accommodate 354 children. It replaced the Hampstead School which had become overcrowded after receiving children from the MAB's idiot asylums at Caterham and Leavesden. By performing such a role, Darenth, from its inception, acted as a school with close ties to asylums and those that had been confined in them. It was supposed to receive children that were 'improvable' and that would benefit from the education that it offered. This ideal was not always achieved and by 1887 only 362 of the 600 children on the site received some form of education.[13] Darenth evidently functioned both as school and asylum.

By moving beyond the asylum as the place of care for the insane it is important to examine how special education also developed as a branch of the mainstream school system. The first special school for those with difficulties learning was founded in Leicester in 1892 by the School Board in the city. Later that same year the London School Board established its first special school and by 1896 there were 24 similar schools in the capital that received 900 children. The children that attended the school in Leicester represented an important milestone. Not only did they attend the first special school in the country, but also they were selected by lay observers, rather than by medical professionals. In contrast the London School Board retained a medical officer to certify the mental incapacity of the children that attended its schools.[14] The differing approaches offered by Leicester and London were evident at the time and not without a degree of friction. With the Leicester School's Inspector stating 'we say in Leicester, that in London the child is sent away, and not taken care of by the Board, but the Leicester Board does take care of him. The London Board deals with him in another direction.'[15] We can see that outside of the capital the reliance on medical opinion and custodial institutions was sneered at. The Leicester experience allowed the child to receive an education and also remain with their family. These responses to the mentally deficient, however, occurred due to local initiatives in the national vacuum that existed until 1899.

Like the school boards in Leicester and London the board in Birmingham pre-empted the legislation of 1899 and offered its own classes for defective children from 1898. The children that attended in Birmingham, like Leicester, were selected by lay observers and consequently we can observe a shift away from the medical sphere in identifying the mentally impaired child, at least outside of the capital.[16] A feature of the provision in Birmingham was that the classes for those with learning difficulties took place in a mainstream infant school and not a separate institution. This attempt at inclusive education reinforces the patchwork approach to those with mental impairments that existed at the end of the nineteenth century.

A consequence of this disparate approach was that education of the mentally ill or disabled child was not a priority in all regions. In Manchester the school boards provided no education for those with learning difficulties and they were forced to remain in mainstream classes until the 1899 legislation.[17] In the late 1890s, an inspection of 40,000 school children in the Manchester area found that there were 525 that could benefit from specialised provision.[18] But day schools for the learning disabled were not developed in Lancashire until after 1899. The management of children with mental incapacities in the education system remained firmly rooted in local enthusiasm and concern. By 1899 the picture was of 1300 children in 31 special schools across England.[19] These tended to be found in large towns and cities, mainly because County Councils did not gain control of education until Local School Boards were abolished by the 1902 Education Act. In rural areas the elected nature of the boards meant that they were ineffective and special education consequently developed much slower.

The impact that these schools had on the lives of individual children that had suddenly been identified as intellectually inferior, and thus different to their peers, is difficult, but also important, to explore. Some brief glimpses are offered through the experiences of children confined in asylums though. On 1 May 1897 William Hill was taken to the Colney Hatch Asylum diagnosed as an imbecile. At his admission he had the mental capacity to state that 'I would never go to school because the boys taunted me'.[20] This is a rare instance where we were able to access the voice of the child and it demonstrates the burden that schooling placed upon some individuals. Hill, confined in an asylum towards the end of our period, did not fit the construction of child insanity that was presented in the earlier chapters. He had the ability to converse and there was no comment recorded in his casefile about him having the appearance of an idiot or imbecile. Rather, it might be assumed that his inability to display mental capacities similar to the other children in his school and his experience of bullying might have made him a distraction in class and he was confined to maintain order. We thus get an image of a child that had their everyday happiness, well-being, and liberty challenged because he had been socially 'othered' by the developing education system. In this case we also meet a child that was confined in an asylum that would have most likely been better managed elsewhere.

Educating the 'Uneducable'

On 10 October 1898, Sir Douglas Galton, a cousin of the pioneering eugenicist Francis Galton, argued at a meeting of the British Child Study Association that 'scientific methods should be devised which would enable school authorities to determine the status of each child in the school'.[21] The following year witnessed the introduction of legislation to meet these demands. How this provision for those with special educational needs developed and how it related to the asylums that still operated alongside them is essential to the analysis here. A core question is why did some children receive education in schools while others experienced confinement in asylums? An explanation is provided by the changing nature of psychiatric nomenclature during the period.

As mentioned earlier the growing importance of eugenicist ideas influenced how the mental health conditions of children were constructed in the asylum. It is now essential to examine how these concepts affected and determined the position of children that remained outside of these institutions. The eugenicist focus on eradicating perceived imperfections meant that those with mental disabilities came under more intense scrutiny than ever before. Francis Galton argued that 'Eugenics co-operates with the workings of Nature by securing that humanity shall be represented by the fittest races'.[22] The mainstream acceptance of these views affected how the 'sub-normal' child was treated. Galton went on to argue that 'what nature does blindly, slowly, and ruthlessly, man may do providently, quickly, and kindly'.[23] Such social Darwinist ideas meant that the identification and classification of the mentally deficient became an issue critical to the survival of civilised society.

The increased visibility of children with difficulties learning in schools, in combination with eugenic ideas, led to more comments on their potential abilities, or lack of them, and a reclassification of the terminology for those with mental disabilities. Commonly used terms such as 'idiocy', 'feeble-minded', and 'weak-minded', that had been deployed interchangeably earlier in the nineteenth century, all developed specific meanings and came to signify various gradations of mental ability by the beginning of the twentieth century.[24] We have already discussed how the language of insanity inside asylums developed but it is also important to judge how it evolved outside of the institution. The change in terminology was significant. The first recorded use of the term 'feeble-minded' was by the controversial civic servant Sir Charles Trevelyan in 1875 when he appealed for an improvement for the education of these individuals. By 1913, and the Mental Deficiency Act, this gradation of disability was to be segregated from society.[25] At the end of the nineteenth century, Mark Jackson argued that feeble-mindedness represented a dangerous borderland between those that could be described as intellectually normal and idiocy.[26] Those that occupied this 'borderland' were thought prone to criminality, poverty, and promiscuity, and consequently posed a threat to society in general. Consequently, concerns were raised about children who displayed feeble-minded tendencies and it was important to regulate their behaviour.

Within this eugenic-influenced reclassification, idiocy was considered the lowest form of mental disability and feeble-mindedness a higher grade of mental capacity that might be remedied with specialised education. In the institutions examined throughout this book it might have been that differing forms of mental disability were filtered in accordance with these labels. However, the management of insanity was never so teleological. Despite the evolving classifications and definitions at an intellectual level the terminology remained fluid and subjective operationally. Evidence for such subjectivity can be found with the children admitted to asylums. Amongst these there were four admitted from the Darenth School and an additional two from schools in Enfield and Feltham. Up until 1891 schooling still came at a price and it has been argued that parents and magistrates were reluctant to force attendance in some cases, hence only six admissions from schools might have been a consequence of children slipping through the administrative cracks in the system.[27] Alternatively, schools were not residential for the working class, so those identified as requiring institutional care were most probably admitted from the home or workhouse and not an educational sphere. The diagnoses given to the children that were sent from schools were: from Darenth an idiot boy transferred to Northamptonshire Asylum in 1888; two imbeciles (one male in 1886 and one female in 1895) to Colney Hatch; and an epileptic boy to Colney Hatch in 1883.[28] The information recorded is sparse, but it was stated that Sydney Wright, aged thirteen and epileptic, was 'very strange in manner' and 'says that after a fit he must kill somebody'.[29] It can be safely assumed that he was removed to Colney Hatch for the protection of the other children confined at Darenth. From the other two schools, John Hook was admitted to the Three Counties Asylum from Enfield as an imbecile, in 1881, and Edward Woods was taken to Colney Hatch from the school in Feltham diagnosed as an epileptic.[30] From the diagnoses of idiocy, imbecility, and epilepsy it can be seen that these children would have suffered conditions so severe that they were unable to be educated and required management in a more regulatory environment. This fits with the changing terminology and as expected we see the lowest gradations of mental disability confined in the asylum.

As well as accepting children from schools, asylums also distributed those that it discharged to them. There were twelve children, all from Colney Hatch and all male except for one, that were sent, in accordance with the view of the Leicester School's Inspector, to Darenth. These were made up of seven imbeciles, two idiots, one epileptic, one melancholic, and one child suffering from mania. Epilepsy featured as an underlying complication in four of these cases. The diagnoses of those children sent to Darenth demonstrate that the language of mental disability vacillated in practice. It would be expected that only those with mild or temporary afflictions would be candidates for education and these children were potentially moved to free up space on asylum wards. No other schools feature in the Discharge Registers of the asylums, suggesting that the special classes and schools in operation were unsuitable for asylum children.

The Darenth School can be thought of as an extension of asylum provision. It was administered as part of the Metropolitan Asylum Board and operated as such, rather than as a special school. Presented as an educational institution, its relationship with asylums demonstrates that diagnosis was not important in the process of selection. The mental conditions of those that attended special schools are more difficult to assess. Places were offered by lay observers on the basis of perceived educative ability so we lose the medical lens used to observe the mentally impaired child. We can assume that the children who found their way to special schools managed to achieve some education, mainly because these institutions were still finding their feet and needed to establish some authority over these conditions. Also we see fewer mild cases of mental disability being sent to asylums, which suggests they were being dealt with through alternative means.

The outlet of a custodial and supposed educational institution, like Darenth, was a luxury that did not extend beyond the capital city in the nineteenth century. In rural areas, the asylum or workhouse remained the only places beyond the domestic sphere that housed the mentally disabled child. Louisa Twining, a Poor Law Guardian in London and child welfare campaigner, commented in 1894 on a 'striking anomaly, and ask[ed] why our poor country children are denied the advantages granted to those of the metropolis'.[31] Such a situation is evident in the admission books of the rural asylums examined here. Bernard Perry, aged twelve, was admitted to the Northamptonshire Asylum on 26 February 1903; he was 'sent from school as unable to learn'.[32] At the Three Counties Asylum, Alice Popper, aged four, was admitted because the 'school mistress says she can teach her nothing'.[33] The children that were unable to progress in schools were at best invisible to their teachers and at worst a cause of nuisance, disruption, and a loss of income to those on a pay-by-results contract. Their inability to be educated also demonstrated a future inability to seek and gain employment and by extension the potential future burden they posed to rate-paying society.

In the late-nineteenth century schooling became an important provision for dealing with those that earlier in the period may have been certified as insane and confined in asylums. Special schools had the goal of observing, developing, and advancing the intellectual capacities of children that had previously been considered incapable of improvement. The records for schools in London and Birmingham reveal a high demand for places, but regional development was uneven. The school board in Manchester made use of philanthropic endeavours, that we will come to in due course, in its approach to special schooling, whilst the rural counties examined were ineffective and failed to provide the same level of provision until after our period ends. Schools did offer an alternative space to manage children suffering from mental ill health or disabilities. As the nineteenth century developed they became crucial sites for identifying those in need of specialist provision. Admissions to asylums from schools were few and this suggests the emergence of a non-medical approach to the identification and treatment of the mentally disabled. It is now important to turn attention to other spaces where children were managed by exploring the development of children's hospitals.

Hospitals for Children

By shifting focus to hospitals we move to another of Victorian England's important institutions of care. From case files of child asylum patients it is immediately apparent that there was little interaction between these two medical provisions. The analysis is thus grounded in locating the place of the mentally impaired child in hospitals generally rather than examining institutional relationships. The hospitals of nineteenth-century England were funded by donations from wealthy benefactors and patrons, and administered by volunteers, trustees, and governors.[34] Those treated inside of them were usually 'a carefully selected group' of the 'deserving' poor that relied on the backing and recommendation of a hospital benefactor.[35] However, during the latter part of the century this requirement began to change as physicians began to place emphasis on medical need over subscriber recommendation.[36] Such a development is exemplified by Andrea Tanner who has demonstrated that by 1891 subscriber recommendations only accounted for 3% of children seen at the Hospital for Sick Children at Great Ormond Street.[37] Even though children were increasingly seen because of their medical needs, the parents and families were still required to pay for, or at least make a contribution towards, the cost of treatment. Consequently, hospitals remained institutions of the 'respectable' working class and out of reach of the most vulnerable in society.[38]

In addition to payment expectations there were clear guidelines about what types of patient should be admitted to hospitals. Children aged under seven were excluded from most along with pregnant women, the infectious, those with venereal diseases, and the insane. Insane children were thus barred because of their age and diagnosis; one exception was Guy's Hospital, London that admitted both the incurable and the insane.[39] The hospital designed specifically for children was a late development in England, mainly due to resistance from the medical establishment. The place for the sick child was thought to be at home, mostly because hospitals were required to raise money from private funds and children were associated with high mortality rates that were detrimental to maintaining a good reputation. Influential figures, such as Florence Nightingale, argued that child deaths often occurred as a result of poor household hygiene and specialised children's hospitals would have had a limited impact on reducing the mortality rate.[40]

It was not until 1852 when the Hospital for Sick Children opened at Great Ormond Street in London and became the first children's hospital in England. To put in perspective the lateness of this development, the *Enfants Malades* had been treating children in Paris for half a century by this point. To maintain a focus on the regions that have been discussed thus far, the Royal Manchester Children's Hospital also opened in 1852 and the Birmingham Children's Hospital was established in 1861. Looking at rural regions, progress was again slower, and the first ward, not hospital, for children was opened at the Northampton General Infirmary in 1889.[41] The development of these provisions for sick children can be viewed in a wider context of childhood starting to be considered as a distinct and separate stage of life from adulthood that required specific expertise to deal with its illnesses. However, those diagnosed with mental impairments were still excluded.

The children's hospital may have come late to England but its ambitions reached beyond the cure of the sick child. Similarly to educational development, the Victorian children's hospital also sought to improve the social standing of the working-class child. The environment, both physical and moral, that these youngsters lived in was considered polluted. So by removing them, at least for a short while, they could be instilled with notions of good hygiene and respectable behaviour that would make them better citizens and also develop ideas of middle-class domesticity among the lower classes.

Despite these lofty goals it is unclear how the hospital accommodated the working-class child suffering from mental illness or disability. Much like the subscriber hospitals of the period, admission to a children's hospital was reliant on the recommendation of a subscriber. David Wright has demonstrated that a similar system operated at the Earlswood Idiot Asylum where working families needed to gain two recommendations.[42] Just like the experience of general hospitals this requirement was not strictly enforced as the period progressed. In fact the children's hospital in Birmingham never required a recommendation. It was founded as a free hospital and aimed to encourage a clientele of the 'deserving' poor through the charging of a small fee for treatment.[43] The shift in focus to medical need was driven by 'physicians seeking advancement and finding its [the hospitals] amenities infinitely preferable to practice in a poor patient's home'.[44] This system, however, was abused at Great Ormond Street where provision for outpatients was accessed by 'persons in a superior position' and subsequently subscriber recommendation remained a part of the admissions process throughout the nineteenth century.[45] The children treated at Great Ormond Street were consequently a privileged group, even if this was not a reflection of their social status.

It is possible to identify the treatment of insanity in children's hospitals by utilising the digital records of these institutions through the Historic Hospital Admission Registers Project (HHARP).[46] This online resource has made admission data available for Great Ormond Street, the Evelina Hospital, and the Alexandra Hospital for Children with Hip Disease, all in London; and the Royal Hospital for Sick Children in Glasgow. For the purpose of this analysis the discussion is restricted to Great Ormond Street and Evelina Hospitals where there were 418 children admitted with diagnoses of mental illness or disability between the years 1852–1907. In comparison with the numbers found in the five asylums this is quite significant. Unfortunately it is not possible to access a wider comparison of the regions investigated here because the records for the Manchester and Birmingham children's hospitals have not survived.

The hospital for children was designed and established to deal specifically with child illnesses, but chronic cases were still excluded from treatment. The diagnoses of all children seen at Great Ormond Street have been examined by Andrea Tanner. She discovered a large number with mental impairments, although she grouped them generically and did not go further by breaking them down into specific diagnoses. Consequently, Tanner found that children with complaints of the 'nervous system' were the third

Table 5.1 Admissions to children's hospitals with a diagnosis of mental illness or disability, 1852–1907

	Great Ormond Street Hospital for Sick Children	*Cromwell House*	*Evelina Hospital*	*Total*
Dementia	28	1	0	29
Epilepsy	166	9	4	179
Idiocy	155	1	24	180
Imbecility	15	0	6	21
Insanity	7	0	0	7
Mania	2	0	0	2
Total	373	11	34	418

Source: http://www.hharp.org/ accessed on 15 January 2014

most recorded group, behind those with ailments linked to the 'joints, bones and muscles' and the 'respiratory system'.[47] Through a manipulation of the HHARP dataset it is possible to extend Tanner's findings and reveal the specific conditions that children were admitted with (Table 5.1).

Please check inserted citation for Table 5.1.Could it change to - Children's hospital admissions for those with a diagnosis of mental illness or disability, 1852-1907 - thanks

It is evident that chronic conditions featured frequently with epilepsy and idiocy being most common. These findings support those of the asylum, in that children with mental disabilities, rather than mental illnesses were most commonly admitted. It also alters understanding of children's hospitals during the period by clearly demonstrating that chronic conditions were regularly treated there. By adopting a wider lens it can be argued that presence of these children in hospitals suggests a broader shift in perceptions of childhood more generally and demonstrates a wider acceptance of childhood being a time that should be cherished and enjoyed amongst nineteenth-century families.

The average age of a child suffering from a mental impairment and admitted to the London children's hospitals was five and a half. This was a considerably younger average than the children admitted to asylums. Meanwhile the gender split was closer to the asylum experience. There were 230 (55%) male admissions and 188 (45%) female. The hospital functioned as a very different arena for treating child mental health than the asylum. Children found themselves confined for much shorter lengths of time. The average duration of stay for those with a mental impairment was twenty-one and a half days. Such a short length of time is a reflec-

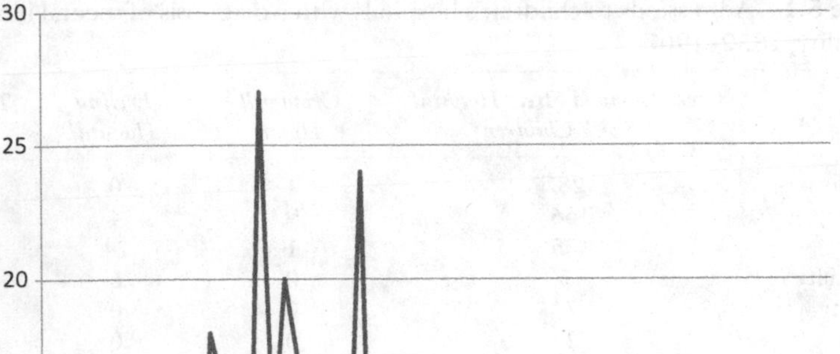

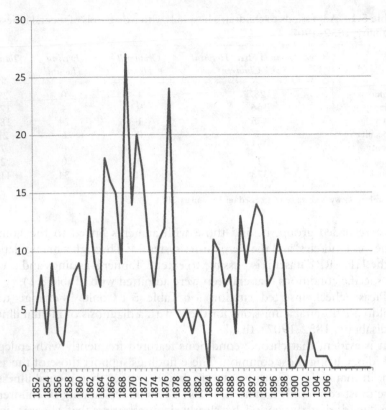

Fig. 5.1 Years of admission to children's hospitals, 1852–1907. *Source*: www.hharp.org accessed 15 January 2014

tion of the hospital's focus on treatment and recovery. Figure 5.1 helps to build a more detailed picture of the hospital's role and demonstrates that the mentally deficient child was admitted to hospitals throughout the period, with the years 1865–1876 seeing the most intensive phase of admissions.

The peaks in hospital admissions occurred earlier than those experienced in asylums. While the asylum encountered more children entering the institutions in 1880s, the peak for hospitals occurred in 1869. Providing an explanation for this disparity requires an exploration of inter-related factors that governed the welfare of children during the period. It may have been caused by the declining importance of subscriber recommendations combined with a degree of unwillingness of families to access the provision of, and social stigma attached to, the asylum. Alternatively, broader socio-economic changes in the distribution of Poor Law medical out-relief might provide the best reasons for difference. Elizabeth Hurren has noted that 1869 was a watershed year in the history of welfare. The circulation of the Goschen Minute signalled the beginning of a 'crusade' against outdoor relief.[48] Consequently, access to medical relief via the Poor Law became more difficult and families with some capacity to pay for treatment sought to bypass the Poor Law. The high-water mark of admissions between the years 1869–1876 certainly fits with such an explanation. An increase in admissions to asylums later in the period might also be explained as a consequence of the Poor Law crusade. Efforts to reduce out-relief had the most impact just as economic downturn set in, especially in agricultural areas; this would have adversely affected the ability of working families to pay for their children's medical care.

Through the admission of children with mental disabilities to hospitals it is possible to identify the networks of care that existed for the mentally ill. Previously Graham Mooney has argued that there was a mixed economy of diagnosis by the mid-nineteenth century. This was represented by the increased hegemony of medical institutions, such as workhouse infirmaries, asylums, and hospitals, in the identification of disease.[49] Again, there is limited understanding of how these diagnostic spaces evolved to accommodate children and the links that existed between them in the management of this shifting population. In previous studies of patient circulation a small overlap has been found in the use of hospital treatment funded by the Poor Law for those that were occasionally dependent on relief.[50] This research, however, only examined medical provision in one region during the eighteenth century. A lack of patient movement between hospitals and asylums here indicates that medical provision for the working class and destitute was distinct and separate by the nineteenth century.

The cohort of child asylum patients contained only one that accessed both asylum and hospital. Kate Steggles was admitted to Great Ormond Street on 22 June 1863, aged six, diagnosed as an epileptic with scarlet fever. The scarlet fever was, however, stated to have been contracted inside the hospital six days after admission. She was then discharged on 11 August 1863, after being a patient for fifty days. Steggles was later admitted to the Three Counties Asylum on 10 November 1866 when aged nine. The uniqueness of the name and the accuracy of the age suggest that this was the same child. Additionally, the Great Ormond Street admission records note that she was admitted from Biggleswade, Bedfordshire; the location from where she was sent to the Three Counties Asylum. In the asylum Steggles was diagnosed as an imbecile, but there was no mention of the epilepsy recorded at the Great Ormond Street hospital, perhaps reflecting the attitudes of doctors to epileptic patients and the creativity of Poor Law Medical Officers in gaining admission. She was discharged from the asylum as recovered on 26 August 1867 only to be readmitted on 31 August 1869. Thereafter she remained until her death on 22 September 1871.[51]

By first accessing the children's hospital it is possible that Steggles had a recommendation from a subscriber. In the years following discharge it appears that circumstances had changed and it is possible that the fortunes of the family altered, which forced them to access the pauper lunatic asylum. Life-cycle causes, such as the incapacitation or death of a carer, were often responsible for triggering admission to the asylum.[52] In this case, however, the family circumstances are unclear. It might have been that Steggles was admitted to Great Ormond Street not because she had received an endorsement, but rather her medical condition piqued the interest of the doctors there. This scenario, however, seems unlikely; epileptics were generally considered unsuitable for hospital care and the scarlet fever that she contracted was common. The experience of Kate Steggles is representative of the exclusivity of the children's hospital. It was clearly a space that accommodated child insanity, but a different type of child was received compared to those confined in asylums. The absence of other cases suggests that hospitals were effective at keeping out those that had previously received relief from the Poor Law. With the large number of children suffering from mental disabilities in hospitals we must assume that care was dependent on social status, rather than medical need.

The unsuitability of the hospital as a site for accommodating child mental disabilities is evident from the comments about them on departure from the London hospitals. The majority of children left with comments such as 'not fit cases', or 'unlikely to improve in the hospital'. It can be seen that the position of the insane child was not secure in children's hospitals, even though they were regularly recorded as patients. There were two children that were recommended by the hospital to be transferred to idiot asylums, one was discharged to an unnamed asylum and the other removed to Earlswood.[53] Additionally there was another child with 'friends' trying to find a place in an idiot asylum for them.[54] The intended destinations of these patients confirm the higher social status of those accessing the hospital, as subscriber recommendation was a requirement for admission to private institutions.[55]

The actions and expectations of the children's families also point towards a different function of the hospital to that of the asylum. Many of the children admitted to asylums were so after a considerable amount of time and usually after the exhaustion of alternative care arrangements. In contrast, John Steer, aged five, from Derby, was diagnosed as an idiot by the Great Ormond Street Hospital and was taken there because 'the father of this boy was so anxious to have an opinion from the hospital'.[56] This example reinforces the view of the children's hospital as a place for the 'respectable' working class. While it is a solitary case and usually medical files, either in the asylum or elsewhere, do not record instances of family thoughts or emotions, we can see that the father sought out the hospital and that he accepted the medical intervention of the doctor in the life of his child.

There was a clear class division between children's hospitals and asylums in caring for those with mental illness or disability. Many of the children admitted to hospitals came from the deserving poor that most likely wanted to avoid the shame of reliance on the Poor Law at all costs. Pauperisation carried a stigma that meant it was not an option resorted to lightly.[57] Such a class divide is problematic when considering the admission of children to asylums presented earlier. Most children dispatched to asylums came from their own homes and were not from destitute families resident in the workhouse. These children therefore were most likely from families that could not afford the cost of medical care, did not have access to a subscriber recommendation, or needed more extensive custodial treatment for a dangerous or destructive child than the hospital could provide. What can be observed is that there were more institutional responses available to the 'respectable' working class for the issue of child insanity than have been considered by the historiography.

Home, Community, and Charity

The Domestic Sphere

Some historians have wrongly assumed that institutional confinement was the 'normal' family response to a mentally disabled child. Such a belief has grown out of Scull's argument that families rushed to admit their mentally impaired members to pauper lunatic asylums.[58] The historian Lynn Hollen

Lees has presented the example of William Turner. In 1885 he was a street trader in London with six children, one of which was 'feeble-minded'. The family was self-supporting and not reliant on parish relief, but in 1887 Turner spoke to Poor Law officials and had his mentally defective son removed to the pauper lunatic asylum. Hollen Lees argues that a 'family obligation to maintain both the very old and the very young was waived in the case of permanent disability'.[59] A situation like Turner's is presented as the norm, but it has been demonstrated in the analysis thus far that this was not the case and families sought to care for children in the home for as long as possible. Domestic and community care arrangements represented important spaces for the long-term care of the insane, but they are also the most difficult to quantify and analyse.[60] Evidence that has survived from the homes of the working poor is extremely rare.[61] The records of asylums provide some insight into the lives and experiences of both the children and their families prior to confinement, but those that never received institutional care remain invisible to the researcher.

Such difficulty in quantifying children in the domestic sphere means it is impossible to accurately say how many children remained outside of the asylum and how they were treated when they did. The records of Poor Law Guardians reveal sporadic mentions of insane pauper children, but they only feature very briefly and usually they were ultimately dispatched to the asylum anyway. Those that never relied on parish assistance are hidden and need to be revealed. One possible way of capturing them is from the decennial census. From 1871 the census conducted across Britain recorded lunatics, idiots, and imbeciles kept in the community. Considering children in the counties where our asylums were located, a consistent picture of recording child mental illness develops and is presented in Table 5.2.

It is clear that child mental ill-health featured on the national census, but it was never recorded in large numbers. The census returns of 1881 reveal that there were 32,717 idiots and imbeciles in England and Wales, 1390 being children in the areas examined in this book. Of these 16,105 were male and 16,612 female, with those over forty-five years old accounting for 9183. These were more than likely misdiagnosed as imbeciles and instead suffered from dementia. On the 1881 census there were only 451 idiots and imbeciles recorded as under the age of five in the whole country.[62] The census obviously has limitations. The quantitative analysis that it allows is restricted to a snapshot of one day in a ten-year period and it excludes those that might be born and subsequently died in intra-census

Table 5.2 Child insanity as a proportion of county populations according to census returns, 1881–1901

	1881	*1891*	*1901*
Beds, Hunts, Herts (Three Counties)	0.02	0.02	0.02
Lancashire	0.02	0.01	0.01
London Area (Colney Hatch)	0.01	0.01	0.02
Northamptonshire	0.02	0.03	0.02
Warwickshire	0.02	0.02	0.02

Note: The data for the 1871 in England is currently unavailable with the archive. The search criteria included children aged thirteen or under at the time of the census, recorded disability as insane, dumb, idiot, or imbecile, and only included first level recorded disabilities

Source: UK Data Archive—Integrated Census Microdata, http://icem.data-archive.ac.uk/, accessed 25–28 May 2014

years. Also it is more than likely that the census has been significantly under-enumerated; a problem that can be effectively demonstrated by returning to child asylum patients.

By taking a 10 % subsample of congenital child patients admitted to the asylums in the years following 1871 and locating them on the census immediately prior to their confinement, the frequency with which their mental health conditions were recorded can be identified. The results of the census analysis indicate that of the patient subsample only 27 % were recorded as being lunatics, idiots, or imbeciles on the census. This is despite the children having suffered from their conditions since birth. Consequently, a picture emerges of parents unwilling to recognise mental defects in their children, a problem that was identified by the contemporary physician Dr George Shuttleworth in 1886.[63] More recently Edward Higgs has argued that lunatics, idiots, and imbeciles outside of the asylum were estimated to have been under-enumerated by as many as a half on the census.[64] The subsample demonstrates that this estimate was optimistic and children were under-enumerated by roughly 75 %. Consequently, we develop a picture on both a specific and general scale of the difficulty in identifying children that never received institutional care. To gain a better understanding of family methods of coping and how children were treated beyond medical and state institutions we explore the role and impact of charity during the period.

Philanthropy

As the nineteenth century progressed the growing influence of middle-class philanthropy increasingly affected, both positively and negatively, the lives of poor children and their families. Hugh Cunningham has argued that 'reformers and philanthropists were deeply imbued with the romantic belief that childhood should be happy, the best time of life, something to which one would look back later both with nostalgia and for inspiration'.[65] A consequence of this romantic view of childhood was a discourse that emerged that began to see the residential space of the family as a home, in a modern sense, for the first time.[66] Some scholars have considered such attitudes towards the homes of working people as a tactic of class differentiation, adopted by the middling sorts in order to distance themselves from working families.[67] It was during this period that the family was ideally supposed to consist of a wage-earning father and a wife working at home, although this model was rarely achieved among the complex and at times extended families of the working class.[68] In such domestic arrangements the welfare of children was solely the concern of women in the household. Philanthropists considered intervention important because they viewed the homes of the poor as the places that contaminated the health and morals of the young. They thought the poor to be indecent and their vices a danger not just to their offspring, but to the fabric of English society in general.

In order to stem such a slide into degeneration it was suggested by activists such as Octavia Hill that middle-class female philanthropists should befriend working-class families and then guide them in correct morals and behaviour.[69] In this discourse children were considered and treated as victims of 'the cruelty of their parents and neighbours'.[70] The emergence of eugenics also meant that the bad heredity of poor families was regularly included as a contributing factor to the mental defects that occurred in children of the poor. Pauperism was viewed as a disease by the philanthropic class and if they did not attempt to contain it then it would inevitably spread to others.[71] This fed the middle-class opinion that the urban poor 'lived like animals, overcrowded, disorganised, fatalistic, without prospect of improvement'.[72] The consequence of such perceptions was that for much of the period middle-class charity relied on the view that urban populations could only survive through individual prudence and industry.[73] These core philanthropic values of self-help and individualism meant that charity was often restricted to those unable to help themselves such as orphans, lunatics, the elderly, and crippled.

Consequently, the under-privileged child became the subject for and symbol of the need for charitable help. Cunningham pinpointed the year 1866 when philanthropic efforts shifted from evangelical work designed to improve the position of children to endeavours aimed at rescuing them from vice-infested working-class communities.[74] This year marked the establishment of Lord Shaftesbury's training ships for boys, a severe outbreak of cholera, economic depression, and the arrival of both the famous child rescuer Thomas Barnardo and William Booth, the founder of The Salvation Army, to London. The scale of philanthropy during this period was certainly staggering. Ellen Ross has noted that in 1885 donations made to charities in London exceeded the national budgets of countries such as Portugal, Sweden, and Denmark.[75] Of these charities there were numerous organisations such as the National Society for the Prevention of Cruelty to Children (1889), Barnardos Homes (1867), the Church of England Waifs and Strays Society (1881), the Society of St Vincent de Paul (1847) who helped Roman Catholic children, numerous homeless missions and shelters, and Ragged Schools (1844) that focused specifically on the children of the poor. These were driven by middle-class men and women who challenged working-class notions of parenting in the late nineteenth century. Eventually they reached the conclusion that the only way poor children could prosper was if they were removed from inadequate parents and living conditions.

'Deserving Objects of Charity'

The mentally defective child provided a specific concern for Victorian philanthropy. The responses to these children were varied and at times reveal the dark underbelly of nineteenth-century charity. Eugenics was again a prominent influence on the philosophies and actions of these groups when it came to the mentally deficient. The National Association for Promoting the Welfare of the Feeble Minded (NAPWFM) was established in 1896 and sponsored by the Charity Organisation Society. The need for such a charity was highlighted by Lord Herschell who stated:

> that above the grade of recognised idiots or imbeciles there was a class of defective beings who without special guidance would be apt to drift into immorality and crime, and it was again to the State to diminish the number of paupers and criminals.[76]

Such a statement demonstrates the shifting understanding of learning disability, at certain levels of society, as discussed throughout this book. Herschell's comments were given medical legitimacy by the noted physician Sir James Creighton, who stated that the 'decrease of infantile mortality that had taken place in recent years tended to the survival of the unfit, and consequently the number of defective children to be dealt with would probably increase rather than diminish'.[77] To tackle their concerns about the feeble-minded the NAPWFM had two core aims: the first was 'the improvement of the physical and mental condition of children so far deficient as to need special care though not actually imbecile; and (2) the kindly supervision of feeble-minded adults in suitable occupations as to save them from degradation.'

Initially the NAPWFM managed homes for feeble-minded girls from Poor Law schools and aimed to protect them from social vices by training them into employment, primarily completing manual domestic tasks.[78] Despite a declared goal of protecting the welfare of the feeble-minded the NAPWFM were enthusiastic about segregation believing that individuals dealt with by the Poor Law were 'constantly leaving the shelter of the workhouse to go into the world, where they are a source of evil and danger to the community'.[79] Consequently, cottage homes were established in London and a steam laundry in Hendon specifically for the confinement and employment of feeble-minded women. The focus of the NAPWFM spanned the age range and the society concerned itself with the welfare of feeble-minded adults socially, as well as the care of children. Following the Education (Defective and Epileptic Children) Act 1899, the NAPWFM began to work with school boards across the country to help provide instruction for feeble-minded children.[80]

The NAPWFM operated at a national level, but there were also regional responses from other individuals and organisations. The lack of provision for those with learning difficulties in Manchester stirred Mary Dendy into action. She was a middle-class reformer and in 1898 founded the Lancashire and Cheshire Society for the Permanent Care of the Feeble-Minded. Its goal was to offer a 'permanent' residential environment for feeble-minded children in the north-west. Consequently, care and control intertwined with some limited education and instruction at the school, established in 1902, at Sandlebridge, Cheshire. Dendy's society and school more explicitly addressed wider social concerns about the feeble-minded and their perceived 'uncontrolled' sexuality.[81] The school initially took thirty feeble-minded children from the Manchester Board Schools. In the wake of the Education (Defective and Epileptic Children) Act it became an official residential school for the feeble-minded of the Manchester Schools Board and thus fulfilled part of their entitlement to those in need of special educational needs.[82] The development of these schools shows the existence of alternative space for children with mental health problems emerging in the north-west of England.

Ellen Pinsent took up a similar cause in Birmingham. She worked within the boundaries of the Birmingham Schools Board, and became a member of the Committee for Special Schools. She was stirred into action by the low levels of attendance in the Board's special schools. Pinsent undertook a programme of inspection for ordinary schools and selected children to be placed in special classes in the city.[83] Pinsent and Dendy both provide examples of the influence local reformers could have during the period. They became responsible, at an individual level, for the selection criteria applied to children in need of special education and they also both became members of the state system to improve education for children with learning difficulties.[84] As the period progressed the importance of lay reformers in the identification and selection processes of children with mental disabilities was evident. Such a situation highlights the broad and complex social context that child mental impairment existed in by the end of the nineteenth century.

Children's Charities

Aside from charities established specifically for the improvement of the mentally defective, there were those, mentioned above, that dealt with children generically. These charities used a variety of approaches to help the children of the Victorian poor, such as shelters, employment, orphan homes, and emigration. Of these strands of assistance, emigration of pauper children to various corners of the British Empire is one that is most eye-catching. The children that were selected for such a fate usually had been filtered through the various elements of a charity before the option of emigration was presented to them. Despite catering for those that were considered not to be mentally impaired they inevitably came into contact with children suffering from mental illness or disability.

Child emigration has a history that predates the Victorian period. As early as 1619 the London Common Council sent 100 children to the Jamestown settlement in Virginia and earlier in the nineteenth century the Children's Friends Society and Ragged School Movement both emigrated children to Australia. The emigration programmes that emerged in the late nineteenth century were often organised along religious lines, although Roman Catholic schemes were often reactions to the fear of proselytising Catholic youths by Protestant organisations. Emigration provided an effective way to settle the empire and at the same time instil bourgeois middle-class values on the working poor. It was as Joy Parr stated 'a safety valve for internal disorder and a path to salvation'.[85] The published motives of the charities themselves reveal a dual purpose for emigration. The Manchester and Salford Boys' and Girls' Refuge stated in 1886: 'we feel we cannot do better for any children that come under our care than to place them in good farm homes in the great Dominion of Canada'.[86] Altruistic as this might appear it was followed by the more expedient comment that 'in no way can destitute children with healthy bodies and sound minds be so cheaply and effectively provided for'.[87] Expense, like elsewhere in this book, was at the forefront of concerns for dealing with these children. The latter statement also highlights an important issue that needs to be explored in further detail and that is the belief that children emigrated from Britain were of 'sound mind'.

The good health of the child was vital to the emigration process. Children were sent to live and work on farms in Canada and thus needed to be able to cope with arduous manual labour. Although the mentally disabled child was on occasion employed in the asylum, it was in a controlled environment and under some form of specialist supervision, a very different work context from the under-populated agricultural regions of the Empire. The children that were sent raised concerns amongst Canadian contemporaries about the export of 'bad heredity' to the Dominion. The Canadian alienist Charles K. Clarke campaigned to have medical checks introduced for immigrants on their arrival to the dominion.[88] The medical examinations that took place in England were not always stringent and emigration was occasionally used by the Manchester and Salford Boys' and Girls' Refuge to dispose of children displaying mental health issues.[89] For example, Fanny R. was noted to have been 'troubled with fits' and consequently passed through ten foster homes because 'no one will put up with her';[90] Eliza M. was described as 'feeble-minded' and returned to Manchester;[91] Edith A. was placed in a hospital for the insane;[92] and Theodore B. was admitted to the insane asylum at Kingston, Ontario in 1905.[93] Such a response to insane children from individuals in England demonstrates a darker side to the philanthropy of the late nineteenth century. Emigration was used as a convenient way of removing mentally disabled children from the Manchester area. It is unclear if the same was true for other regions. The children sent from The Refuge in Manchester were regularly sent to Canada through a scheme operated by Dr Thomas Barnardo. This initially saw them escorted in the migration process with prominent agents that ran distribution homes in Canadian provinces, such as Maria Rye and Annie MacPherson. From 1880, however, Barnardo took more direct control over the practice. It appears, at least on the face of it, that the children sent from London and examined by different Medical Officers did not display evidence of mental ill-health.

Furthermore evidence from the Middlemore Emigration Homes in Birmingham suggests that children with mental illnesses or disabilities were not sent to Canada from the city. The Refuge in Manchester and Barnardos in London provided a multitude of institutional options for the care of destitute children, but the Middlemore Homes only dealt with emigration and thus its reputation relied on sending good stock. Between the years 1872 and 1948 they sent over 5000 children to Canada. The records show that the homes had some dealings with insane children, however these were extremely limited and the nature of illness is somewhat vague. For example, William Howell was returned from Canada in 1876 because he was 'incorrigible' and was later described as 'not a bad boy but peculiar'.[94] Matilda Jackson, aged twelve, was admitted to the home in July 1874 in order to be sent to Canada but was later 'dismissed as insane'.[95] It appears therefore that emigration was used as a particular means for dealing with the mentally defective in Manchester and not in the other areas examined here. The regional nature of provision for children in the late nineteenth and early twentieth centuries is thus reinforced through this philanthropic experience.

As well as emigration programmes, Barnardos operated a number of residential homes and institutions for children both physically and mentally disabled and in need of some degree of care. Thomas Barnardo began work in London in 1867 and opened up his first home for boys in 1870 in Stepney.[96] In the areas that were home to the five asylums Barnardos established the Dallington Lodge in Northampton in 1902 that was a home for girls with special educational needs (after 1933 it became available to both sexes). There was also a home in Birkdale, Lancashire, for the general care of sick children, as well as various homes situated across London. It is not clear whether the insane were managed in these homes as their records have not survived. Nevertheless the impact of philanthropy in the late nineteenth century demonstrates that there was broad social concern about children suffering from mental illness and disability. In turn various spaces emerged to accommodate children. Many of these took traditional forms, such as residential schools and workhouses, but there was also the introduction of new methods of managing the insane child. These were homes for the mentally defective operated by charities and the emigration of children, the latter representing the most extreme of these alternative spaces.

The relationship between the spaces of caring for insane children and the asylum are of importance. It helps to build an understanding of how the various elements of care fit together within a mosaic of provision and whether the care of these children was part of a broader system of care or whether charities and asylums operated independently. Only one child was admitted to our asylums from charitable institutions. That was Thomas Burcombe, admitted to Colney Hatch in 1899, from the Barnardo's home in Stepney.[97] There were no children discharged to the care of charities from our asylums. The spaces of care for insane children appear therefore to be distinct and separate. The philanthropic endeavours that sought to confine the insane would have no need to resort to the asylum and would carefully select their children for admission. Whereas the more general charities appear not to have had contact with asylums, either dealing with insane children in their own ways, such as the Manchester Refuge, or choosing not to deal with the insane child at all and leaving their welfare for others such as the Poor Law and specialist charities.

Conclusion

The issue of child insanity intersects with a wide and varied literature of childhood, education, health, disability, charity, and empire. We have seen that mentally deficient children were dealt with in a variety of spaces and places. Child insanity was a much more important and universal issue than has been acknowledged and its impact extends beyond the asylum and Poor Law to the core of nineteenth-century society. The development of alternative spaces for insane children was part of a wider trend in the development of social spaces to observe and control children. Such an expansion emerged from the recognition of children as individuals in their own right and in need of guidance and direction for both individual and social development. Schools became key locations to observe the child and hospitals were used to better understand the illnesses of children. The discussion here has demonstrated that philanthropy became a tool to identify and shift the problem of child mental illnesses. What stands out is that nineteenth-century society developed responses to childhood illness that clearly separated it from the adult world.[98] Such segregation not only occurred by age, but also by health with the able-bodied filtered out from the perceived deficient and weak.

The motives of each of the alternative spaces that dealt with the mentally defective child are important and varied. The introduction of schools sought to improve the intellectually incapable and eventually led to the school becoming the site for the identification of childhood health defects. The Children's Hospital provided medical care and unlike the asylum did not act as an institution of custody and control. Philanthropy served a dual purpose; it sought the improvement of the child but also removed the mentally inferior child that was beyond help.

The chapter highlights how children were segregated by mental ability before the introduction of the Mental Deficiency Act 1913. Schools, hospitals, and philanthropy, as well as asylums, all identified and separated the child suffering from some form of mental incapacity from society. This separation was not always physical, like the schools of Darenth or Sandlebridge or the emigration programmes of the north-west, but was about creating an imagined divide. A core feature was the construction of the child with learning difficulties as 'the other' and highlighting their mental differences to peers, family, and society as a whole.

The treatment of children with mental illnesses or disabilities also sits within a wider discourse about the idea of the family during this time. Cunningham has argued that in the late nineteenth century there was a growing sense that working families were either not facing up to their responsibilities towards children or were incapable of looking after them properly.[99] Displaying the interconnectivity of the issues at the heart of this chapter the establishment of elementary education had a wider goal of instilling 'morality, and patriotism, and to train children in regular habits'.[100] The state had therefore appropriated the role and authority in the development of children that had previously been held by the family.

We can see that in order to better understand the nature of child insanity it is important to look away from the institution of the asylum and take in wider avenues of care. Whereas most scholars have focused on the asylum as the primary locus of care for the insane, the range of spaces occupied by child mental disability demonstrate that this was not the case.[101] When the literature has attempted to move outside of the asylum the analysis has been too narrow and mostly concentrated on the domestic sphere.[102] The analysis here demonstrates that the spaces and places for dealing with the insane child were varied and worthy of more detailed examination. In short this book introduces new unexplored avenues of debate that build on the analysis conducted in the asylum and questions the current understanding of how children, not just the insane, were considered and treated during the second half of the nineteenth century and early twentieth century.

Notes

1. See the collection of essays in P. Bartlett and D. Wright (eds.), *Outside the Walls of the Asylum: The History of Care in the Community 1750–2000* (London: Athlone, 1999); Also: A. Suzuki, 'The Household and the Care of Lunatics in Eighteenth Century London,' in P. Horden and R. Smith (eds.), *The Locus of Care*, pp. 153–17; and A. Suzuki, 'Enclosing and Disclosing Lunatics within the Family Walls: Domestic Psychiatric Regime and the Public Sphere in Early Nineteenth-Century England,' in Bartlett and Wright (eds.), *Outside the Walls*, pp. 115–131.
2. T. Lacqueur, 'Working Class Demand and the Growth of English Elementary Education,' in L. Stone (ed.), *Schooling and Society* (Baltimore: Johns Hopkins University Press, 1978), p. 193; E. Hopkins, *Childhood Transformed: Working-Class Children in Nineteenth-Century England* (Manchester: Manchester University Press, 1994), p. 233.
3. J. Humphries, *Childhood and Child Labour in the British Industiral Revolution* (Cambridge: Cambridge University Press, 2010), pp. 310–312; Humphries, 'Childhood and Child Labour in the British Industrial Revolution,' *The Economic History Review*, 66/2 (2013), pp. 395–418.
4. Humphries, *Childhood and Child Labour*, p. 365; H. Cunningham, *Children and Childhood in Western Society since 1500* (London: Longman, 1995), p. 102.
5. Hopkins, *Childhood Transformed*, p. 237.
6. D. Pritchard, *Education of the Handicapped, 1760–1960* (Abingdon: Routledge, 1963), p. 116.
7. Hopkins, *Childhood Transformed*, p. 246.
8. D. Wright, '"Childlike in his Innocence": Lay Attitudes Towards "Idiots" and "Imbeciles" in Victorian England,' in D. Wright and A. Digby (eds.), *From Idiocy to Mental Deficiency: Historical Perspectives on People with Learning Disabilities* (London: Routledge, 1996), pp. 118–133; A. Digby and P. Searby, *Children, School and Society in Nineteenth-Century England* (London: The Macmillan Press, 1981), p. 13.
9. A. Davin, 'Imperialism and Motherhood,' *History Workshop Journal*, 5 (1978), pp. 9–65.

10. Hopkins, *Childhood Transformed*, p. 247.
11. S. Wright, 'Moral Instruction, Urban Poverty and English Elementary Schools in the Late Nineteenth Century,' in N. Goose and K. Honeyman (eds.), *Childhood and Child Labour in Industrial England: Diversity and Agency, 1750–1900* (Farnham: Ashgate, 2013), pp. 227–296, p. 295.
12. Pritchard, *Education of the Handicapped*, p. 115.
13. Pritchard, *Education of the Handicapped*, p. 58.
14. P. Potts, 'Medicine, Morals and Mental Deficiency: The Contribution of Doctors to the Development of Special Education in England,' *Oxford Review of Education*, 9/3 (1983), pp. 181–196, p. 182.
15. Cited in Pritchard, *Education of the Handicapped*, p. 122.
16. BCA, SB/B11/1/1/1, Birmingham Education Committee Speical Schools Committee of the School Board Minutes, 10 February 1898–17 March 1903, p. 1; Pritchard, *Education of the Handicapped*, pp. 122–127.
17. 'The Education of Defective Children,' *The Manchester Guardian*, 19 May 1898, p. 12.
18. 'Care of the Feeble-Minded,' *The Manchester Guardian*, 17 October 1898, p. 9.
19. Pritchard, *Education of the Handicapped*, p. 131.
20. LMA, Friern Hospital (Colney Hatch), Male Casebook 44, H12/CH/B/13/044, William Hill, Admission no. 12674, p. 134.
21. 'The Care of Feeble-Minded Children: Address by Sir Douglas Galton,' *The Manchester Guardian*, 11 October 1898, p. 8.
22. F. Galton, *Essays in Eugenics* (London: The Eugenics Education Society, 1909), p. 42.
23. Ibid.
24. A discussion of the contemporary classification is provided by Potts, 'Medicine, Morals, and Mental Deficiency,' p. 184; also J. Goodman, 'Pedagogy and Sex: Mary Dendy (1855–1933), Feeble-Minded Girls and the Sandlebridge Schools, 1902–33,' *History of Education*, 34/2 (2005), pp. 171–187, p. 173.
25. Pritchard, *Education of the Handicapped*, p. 61.
26. M. Jackson, *The Borderland of Imbecility: Medicine, Society and the Fabrication of the Feeble Mind in Late Victorian and Edwardian England* (Manchester: Manchester University Press, 2000).
27. Cunningham, *Children and Childhood*, pp. 103–106.
28. NRO, St Crispin Collection, Out of County Casebook 2, NCLA/6/2/3/2, James Dennis, Admission no., p.; LMA, Friern Hospital (Colney Hatch), Male Casebook 33, H12/CH/B/13/033, Syndey Wright, Admission no. 9149, p. 237; LMA, Friern Hospital (Colney Hatch), Female Casebook 42, H12/CH/B/11/042, Marian Glover, Admission no. 9443, p. 42;

LMA, Friern Hospital (Colney Hatch), Male Casebook 45, H12/CH/B/13/045, Robert Hawkins, Admission no. 12207, p. 267.

29. LMA, Sydney Wright, p. 237.
30. BLA, Three Counties, Male Casebook 6, LF31/6, John Hook, Admission no. 3914, p. 133; LMA, Friern Hospital (Colney Hatch), Male Casebook 38, H12/CH/B/13/038, Edward Woods, Admission no. 10770.
31. 'Idiot Children and Epileptics under the Poor Law,' 24 January 1894, p. 13.
32. NRO, St Crispin collection, Male Patient Casebook 10, NCLA/6/2/1/10, Bernard Perry, Admission no. 5388, p. 155.
33. BLAS, Three Counties, Female Casebook 3, LF29/3, Alice Popper, Admission no. 2589, p. 310.
34. R. Porter, 'The Gift Relation: Philanthropy and Provincial Hospitals in Eighteenth Century England,' in L. Granshaw and R, Porter (eds.), *The Hospital in History* (London: Routledge, 1989), pp. 149–178.
35. J. Reinarz, 'Investigating the "Deserving" Poor: Charity and the Voluntary Hospitals in Nineteenth-Century Birmingham,' in A. Borsay and P. Shapely (eds.), *Medicine, Charity and Mutual Aid: The Consumption of Health and Welfare in Britain, c.1550–1950* (Aldershot: Ashgate, 2007), pp. 111–134, p. 111; Reinarz, *Healthcare in Birmingham: A History of the Birmingham Teaching Hospitals, 1779–1939* (Woodbridge: Boydell & Brewer, 2009).
36. J. Lane, *A social History of Medicine: Health, Healing and Disease in England, 1750–1950* (London: Routledge, 2001), p. 87; E. Lomax, *Small and Special: The Development of Hospitals for Children in Victorian Britain* (London: Wellcome Institute for the History of Medicine, 1996), pp. 8–9; Reinarz, 'Investigating the "Deserving" Poor,' p. 122.
37. A. Tanner, 'Choice and the Children's Hospital: Great Orond Street Hospital and their Families 1855–1900,' in Borsay and Shapely (eds.), *Medicine, Charity and Mutual Aid*, pp. 135–162, p. 142.
38. Lomax, *Small and Special*, p. 79; Reinarz, 'Investigating the "Deserving" Poor,' p. 113; Lane, *Social History of Medicine*, p. 88; Tanner, 'Choice and the Children's Hospital,' p. 144.
39. Lane, *Social History of Medicine*, p. 83.
40. F. Nightingale, *Notes on Nursing: What it is and What it is Not* (London: Duckworth, 1952, first published 1859).
41. F.F. Waddy, *A History of Northampton General Hospital, 1743–1948* (Northampton: Gildhall Press, 1974), p. 46.
42. D. Wright, *Mental Disability in Victorian England: The Earlswood Asylum 1847–1901* (Oxford: Clarendon, 2001).
43. Reinarz, 'Investigating the "Deserving" Poor,' pp. 119–120.
44. Lomax, *Small and Special*, p. 13.
45. *Twenty-Fourth Annual Report of the Hospital for Sick Children* (London, 1876), p. 5.

46. The records are available at www.hharp.org
47. Tanner, *Choice and the Children's Hospital*, p. 152.
48. E. Hurren, 'Belonging, Settlement and the New Poor Law in England and Wales 1870s-1900s,' in S. King and A. Winter (eds.), *Migration, Settlement and Belonging in Europe 1500–1930s: Comparative Perspectives* (Oxford: Berghahn Books, 2013), pp. 127–152, p. 134.
49. G. Mooney, 'Diagnostic Spaces: Workhouse, Hospital, and Home in Mid-Victorian London,' *Social Science History*, 33/3 (2009), pp. 357–390.
50. A. Tomkins, 'Paupers and the Infirmary in Mid-Eighteenth-Century Shrewsbury,' *Medical History*, 43/2 (1999), pp. 208–227.
51. BLA, Three Counties, Admission Register 1, LF27/1, Kate Steggles, Admission no. 1277.
52. C. Smith, 'Living with Insanity: Narratives of Poverty, Pauperism and Sickness in Asylum Records 1840–76,' in A. Gestrich, E. Hurren, and S. King (eds.), *Poverty and Sickness in Modern Europe: Narratives of the Sick Poor, 1780–1938* (London: Continuum, 2012), pp. 117–142.
53. http://www.hharp.org/admissions/fd4fb6c7/29182?item=18, Percy Jones, accessed 03/12/2012; www.hharp.org David Halford was admitted to Earlswood, accessed 15/01/2014.
54. www.hharp.org Bessie Newman, accessed 15/01/2014.
55. David Wright, *Earlswood*.
56. www.hharp.org John Steer, Admitted 29/08/1871, accessed 15/01/2014.
57. Pritchard, *Education of the Handicapped*, p. 57.
58. Scull, *Museums of Madness*.
59. Hollen Lees, 'The Survival of the Unfit: Welfare Policies and Family Maintenance in Nineteenth-Century London,' in P. Mandler (ed.), *The Uses of Charity: The Poor on Relief in the Nineteenth-Century Metropolis* (Philadelphia: University of Pennsylvania Press, 1990), pp. 68–91, p. 69.
60. C. Smith, 'Living with Insanity,' pp. 126–127; N. Tomes, *A Generous Confidence: Thomas Story Kirkbride and the Art of Asylum Keeping, 1840–83* (Cambridge: Cambridge University Press, 1984), p. 109; Wright, 'Familial Care of Idiot Children'; Melling et.al., '"A Proper Lunatic for Two Years": Pauper Lunatic Children in Victorian and Edwardian England. Child Admissions to the Devon County Lunatic Asylum, 1845–1914,' *Journal of Social History*, 31/2 (1997), pp. 371–405.
61. Suzuki, 'Enclosing and Disclosing Lunatics'; Suzuki, *Madness at Home: The Psychiatrist, the Patient and the Family in England, 1820–1860* (Berkeley: University of California Press, 2006).
62. Shuttleworth, *BMJ*, 1886, pp. 183–184.
63. Shuttleworth, *BMJ*, 1886, pp. 183–184.
64. E. Higgs, *Making Sense of the Census: The Manuscript Returns for England and Wales, 1801–1901* (London: Public Record Office, 1989), pp. 74–75.

65. Cunningham, *Children and Childhood*, p. 160.
66. L. Davidoff, *Thicker than Water: Siblings and their Relations, 1780–1920* (Oxford: Oxford University Press, 2012), p. 22.
67. Davidoff and C. Hall, *Family Fortunes: Men and Women of the English Middle Class 1780–1950* (London: Routledge, 2002).
68. H. Bosanquet, *The Family* (London: Macmillan, 1906), p. 222.
69. J. Lewis, 'Family Provision of Health and Welfare in the Mixed Economy of Care in the Late Nineteenth and Twentieth Centuries,' *Social History of Medicine*, 8/1 (1995), pp. 1–16, p. 5.
70. Cunningham, *Children of the Poor*, p. 133.
71. Hollen Lees, 'Survival of the Unfit,' p. 81.
72. P. Mandler, 'Poverty and Charity in the Nineteenth-Century Metropolis: An Introduction,' in Mandler (ed.), *The Uses of Charity*, Introduction, p. 7.
73. Mandler, 'Poverty and Charity,' p. 13.
74. Cunningham, *Children of the Poor*, pp. 134–135.
75. E. Ross, 'Hungry Children: Housewives and London Charity, 1870–1918,' in Mandler, *The Uses of Charity*, pp. 161–196, p. 164.
76. 'The National Association for Promoting the Welfare of the Feeble-Minded,' *British Medical Journal*, 18 June 1898, p. 1617.
77. *BMJ*, ibid.
78. Pritchard, *Education of the Mentally Handicapped*, p. 180.
79. 'National Association for Promoting the Welfare of the Feeble Minded,' *BMJ*, 14 July 1900, p. 100.
80. 'National Association,' *BMJ*, 14 July 1900, p. 100.
81. Goodman, 'Pedagogy and Sex,' p. 172; Pritchard, *Education of the Mentally Handicapped*, p. 181; Jackson, *The Borderland of Imbecility*, p. 67.
82. Pritchard, *Education of the Mentally Handicapped*, p. 181.
83. Ibid., p. 182.
84. A. Brown, 'Ellen Pinsent: Including the 'Feebleminded' in Birmingham, 1900–1913,' *History of Education*, 34/5 (2005), pp. 535–546; Goodman, 'Pedagogy and Sex'.
85. J. Parr, *Labouring Children: British Immigrant Apprentices to Canada, 1869–1924* (London: Croom Helm, 1980), p. 27.
86. MCL, *Annual Report of the Manchester and Salford Boys' and Girls' Refuge*, 1886, p. 14.
87. MCL, *Annual Report of Manchester and Salford Boys' and Girls' Refuge*, 1889, p. 14.
88. I. Dowbiggin, '"Keep this Young Country Sane": C.K. Clarke, Immigration Restriction, and Canadian Psychiatry, 1890–1925,' *Canadian Historical Review*, 76/4 (1995), pp. 598–627, p. 605; also A. Bashford, 'Insanity

and Immigration Restriction,' in C. Cox and H. Marland (eds.), *Migration, Health and Ethnicity in the Modern World* (Basingstoke: Palgrave Macmillan, 2013), pp. 14–35, p. 20.
89. S. Taylor, 'Insanity, Philanthropy and Emigration: Dealing with Insane Children in Late-Nineteenth-Century North-West England,' *History of Psychiatry*, 25/2 (2014), pp. 224–236.
90. GMCRO, Manchester & Salford Refuge, Emigration Files, M189/7/2/3/006.
91. GMCRO, Manchester & Salford Refuge, Emigration Files, M189/7/2/5/009.
92. GMCRO, Manchester & Salford Refuge, Emigration Files, M189/7/2/5/048-54.
93. GMCRO, Manchester & Salford Refuge, Emigration Files, M189/7/3/19/239-241.
94. BCA, Middlemore Emigration Homes, Entrance Book Boys, MS517/472, p. 71.
95. BCA, Middlemore Emigration Homes, Entrance Book Girls, MS517/471, p. 61.
96. http://www.barnardos.org.uk/what_we_do/our_history/history_faqs.htm, accessed 12/02/2014.
97. LMA, Friern Hospital (Colney Hatch), Male Casebook 48, H12/Ch/B/13/048, Thomas Burcombe, Admission no. 13215, p. 80.
98. Tanner, 'Choice and the Children's Hospital,' p. 137.
99. Cunningham, *Children and Childhood*, p. 152.
100. Cunningham, *Children and Childhood*, p. 157.
101. Scull, *Museums of Madness*; Scull, *Most Solitary of Afflictions*.
102. For example see the collection of essays contained in: Bartlett and Wright, *Outside the Walls*; Melling et al., 'Proper Lunatic'.

CHAPTER 6

Conclusion

Nellie Chambers was aged eight when she was taken from her home to the Berrywood Asylum on 31 January 1896. She was diagnosed as an idiot, a disability which she had lived with since birth, and it was noted on her case-file, in a rare instance of emotion, that 'she had sufficient intelligence to feel the parting from her mother'.[1] For this young child it must have seemed inconceivable that she would never live with her family again, and that she would remain in the asylum until she died, at the age of thirty, some twenty-two years later. Three years earlier, Arthur Morecock, also aged eight, had been admitted to the Birmingham Borough Asylum described as a congenital imbecile.[2] Unlike Nellie Chambers, Arthur Morecock had experience of institutional confinement and was transferred to the Birmingham Asylum from the Warwickshire County Asylum at Hatton. He did not, however, share the same fate and found himself discharged back to the Birmingham Poor Law Union Workhouse only five months after admission. Following this transfer we lose sight of Arthur Morecock, but it is difficult to imagine that he had a future where he was not in near contact with state institutions and public assistance. These stories can be seen as particularly emotive, and they invoke our sympathies as a modern observer for a variety of reasons: we see a young girl removed from her family, a boy kept and moved between institutions, an uncertain future, and a death in isolation. However, beyond these emotional connections Chambers and Morecock serve as emblematic examples of the different approaches taken to children by institutions in the nineteenth century.

S.J. Taylor, *Child Insanity in England, 1845-1907*, Palgrave Studies in the History of Childhood, DOI 10.1007/978-1-137-60027-1_6

At this point it is clear that the narratives of the 773 children admitted to the five asylums intersect with a wide and varied historical literature covering topics such as childhood, education, health, disability, charity, and empire. In the preceding chapters we have seen that mentally ill or disabled children were dealt with in a variety of spaces and places. Child insanity was thus a much more important and universal issue than has been acknowledged and its impact extends beyond the asylum and Poor Law to the core of nineteenth-century society. The development of alternative spaces of care and treatment for insane children was part of a wider trend in the development of social spaces to observe and control the young. Such an expansion emerged from the recognition of children as individuals in their own right and in need of guidance and direction for both individual and social development. By the end of the century, schools had established themselves, however unwittingly, as key sites to observe the health of children; and hospitals were increasingly being used to better understand the varied and specific illnesses of the young. In addition to these developments, philanthropy became an important tool to identify and shift the problem of child mental illnesses further afield from the locality. What this book highlights is that nineteenth-century society developed responses to childhood illness that clearly separated it from the adult world.[3] Such segregation was not only defined by age, but also by health with the able-bodied filtered from the perceived deficient and weak.

In this context, historical understandings of children with mental illnesses or disabilities has been narrow and underdeveloped. The experiences of children have either been overlooked or dismissed as domestic issues.[4] Furthermore, the pauper lunatic asylums that were established in the second half of nineteenth-century England have not explicitly been examined as a network of medical institutions. Consequently, the regional nature of admission and treatment means that any extrapolation of studies to a national scale is flawed. At the moment the historiography overemphasises local quirks, overstates variations between institutions examined in different contexts, and simultaneously overlooks nuances in broader typological, regional, and national trends. Against this scholarly backdrop, child patients have been used in this book as a vehicle to better understand asylums. Their institutional experiences have been reconstructed and used to compare the function and purpose of five asylums, in order to evaluate how their management and operation varied according to local needs. By doing so discussions of child insanity have extended here beyond the asylum, turning the spotlight towards a mixed economy of makeshifts that existed for the care of children with mental illness and disability in nineteenth-century society.

Lived Experiences of Child Mental Illness

By understanding how mental impairment in childhood was diagnosed, treated, and managed it has been possible to enhance understandings of children and childhood, more generally, in the nineteenth century. The multi-institutional approach of this book has drawn a more detailed picture of the children confined, highlighted the frequency with which they were admitted, and also shown how they were thought of in comparison to 'normal' or healthy youngsters. A key part of the process was the formulation of a new framework that has allowed access to a new historical perspective about the causes of child mental ill-health during the period. This framework demonstrates the importance of family testimony in the process of diagnosis and emphasises how asylum doctors increased their control of childhood insanity in late-nineteenth-century England. A micro-study of those admitted as idiots provided a specific exploration of the most commonly recorded diagnosis for children. Importantly, this process highlighted the subjectivity and fluidity of child insanity with an underlying friction between the competing medical discourses of the Poor Law and asylum at its heart. In this milieu of medical knowledge the insane child's voice has been particularly difficult to save. But a better developed knowledge of how pauper children were observed by the attendants and medical men responsible for their everyday care was possible. The focus on medical conditions also revealed a fundamental and systematic typological divergence in practice and experience between our asylums, with the rural institutions of Berrywood and Three Counties admitting more children and providing more thorough checks of them once inside the asylum.

Moving on from examinations of children, it has been crucial to locate their experiences of mental illness and childhood across our asylums. Previously, the historical literature has focused either on the grand narrative of insanity and institutional confinement, or on case-studies of single asylums or localities, that provide an element of detail and nuance albeit in isolation.[5] Central to much thinking has been the regulatory role of the asylum, especially for the long-term and congenital insane, such as children. Regional case-studies have introduced local experiences and added texture to the debate. They have also demonstrated that the creation, function, and evolution of asylums occurred in a regional context. These studies have offered a starting point to further analyse the uneven development of asylum provision across the country. The only way to develop a clearer understanding of the 'asylum system' however, was if a number of institutions were critically examined through the same analytical prism for the first time.

By doing so it was discovered that there was a variation in management and care between asylums located in rural and urban areas. It had been assumed that the nineteenth-century phenomena of urbanisation and industrialisation were catalysts for the admission of paupers to asylums.[6] This was not the case for children. Although the impact of urbanisation and industrialisation were driving forces, asylums serving rural areas were more frequently the places where insane child were deposited. The reasons for such divergence were grounded in local attitudes. The asylum in Northamptonshire developed a 'children's block' so it could maximise its income from the confinement of out-county children. Rural asylums however, did not simply function as vacuums for unwanted children. The Berrywood Asylum was much less interested in the admission of local youngsters that incurred an expense to local ratepayers and also commanded a lower fee at the institution.[7] Moreover, the asylums that were situated in large urbanised cities were just one element in a broader mosaic of provision for children and the insane that evolved in those areas.

The empirical and typological differences in the child experience of asylums were matched by the qualitative experience. The city asylums failed to live up to the assumptions of the historiography, and the duration of institutional confinement for children was on average substantially less than their rural counterparts. In turn, the death rates of rural asylums were startlingly high. This was partly because the asylums were long-term destinations for insane children in these areas, but also due to the use of the institution as a hospice for the terminally ill and a consequence of underinvestment in facilities and resources. Outside of the asylum there were few alternatives for the mentally impaired child and work opportunities accessible to them in adult life were limited, especially considering the downturn in agriculture from the 1870s. Hence, one might draw parallels with Scull's argument about asylums being nothing more than 'warehouses of the unwanted'. When one looks deeper the evidence does not, however, support such conclusions. The rural asylums did not just leave children to waste away but attempted to better understand their illnesses and disabilities. Also, it found vocations for them inside the asylum and thus demonstrated their productivity in a controlled setting.

It can be said with confidence that the asylum network was not uniform or standardised in its approaches and responses to children. Experiences varied significantly between the urban and rural. We can now start to think of the asylum as part of a medical landscape that existed for the care of the insane child. Within this setting the role of the asylum as either a magnet that pulled children into the institution or a pump that circulated them to alternative provisions has been examined. This further confirmed the differing roles of urban and rural asylums. This is an important issue. Where local studies of single institutions have been conducted it is now important to try and locate them within this broader typological theme of functionality. For example, can similar hypotheses be supported in all rural and urban settings? Or was the use of the asylum more nuanced than these parameters and does the institution need to be regionally deconstructed further? These are important questions that will have to be taken in future research.

It is accurate to say that child mental health was an important social issue of the nineteenth century that led a number of diverse medical and social responses. For a variety of reasons these children have been considered from a medical or care-giver perspective, although there are now increasing attempts to locate individual experience and the voice of the child. The new places and spaces introduced that both defined and dealt with children that were mentally impaired have extended discussions beyond the boundaries of medical responses and into new debates about both the care of the insane and children in nineteenth-century England. Consequently, the argument about the management of the mentally ill or disabled child has moved beyond institutions designed for the reception of the insane and into the fabric of nineteenth-century medical and welfare provision for the poor. By the end of the century, with the increased influence of the eugenics movement, the lexicon of insanity had also been modified. Those labelled idiots, imbeciles, feeble-minded or weak-minded, either as a result of medical or lay diagnosis, were not only more visible to the rest of society, but were also targets of moral judgements about their behaviour. With increased awareness came more varied responses and greater impetus for dealing with insane children. Many new avenues of care were offered by private philanthropy, and the emigration of children suffering from mental disabilities was a major change that has not yet been adequately discussed or debated.[8]

We now have a more complete understanding of the types of children confined in asylums and how these institutions functioned within a wider system of care. A number of themes have also been uncovered that had not, up until now, been explored: such as the urban asylum as a place to circulate rather than confine the insane, the apparent trade in child patients, and the emigration of the mentally impaired. These conclusions have introduced new thinking to the debate about the function of pauper lunatic asylums and methods to deal with the insane, and it is hoped that future scholarship will drive the discussion into even more diverse medical and social contexts.

While the histories of asylums and insanity have featured heavily, it is evident that the experience of children admitted to pauper lunatic asylums in the second half of the nineteenth century sits at a large and broad historiographical intersection that encompasses the histories of psychiatry, asylums, childhood, disability, welfare, and migration. Most obviously, questions about how childhood was experienced between the years 1845 and 1907 by children with mental health issues have been asked. For instance, when Ellen Ridings was described as 'a demented little idiot' on her admission to the Prestwich Asylum, in 1885, it appears that rather than being a medical description, this was a value laden judgement that labelled the child.[9] The medical nomenclature of 'demented', meaning to have lost mental faculty, combined with idiot, those assumed to have never had mental faculty, suggests that Ridings was demeaned on her entry to the asylum—she, in essence, was no longer a child, but in fact a 'demented little idiot'. The interaction between children and a number of specialised institutions occurs at a time when specific and distinct discourses about childhood were being shaped and applied. A general conclusion would be that childhood for the mentally ill or disabled was an experience of segregation from families and communities. This isolation manifested itself in a number of forms. Most obviously through the institutional confinement of children in the asylum, but also through the 'othering' of the insane child deemed inferior to their peers, and in the most extreme sense the physical removal of the child from the country.

In line with contemporaneous applications, the conceptualisation of the 'innocent' Victorian childhood by historians has not accommodated the mentally ill or disabled. Hugh Cunningham argued that the late-nineteenth century saw the beginnings of the modern idea of a sheltered and romantic childhood that removed the child from the adult world.[10] The embodiment of this separation, Cunningham states, was the introduction of elementary education. Schools symbolised the end of the child as an economic asset. It is, of course, difficult to include the children admitted to asylums in such a discourse. Their very presence meant that they were judged to be incapable of education, the central pillar of the modern idea of childhood, and they regularly fulfilled economic roles in asylums, while segregated from their families and communities in adult institutions. Moving beyond the asylum, children that were emigrated were sent to Canada not for rest or recuperation, but they provided manual labour on rural farms in conditions far worse than experienced in England.[11] Thus the insane child held an economic role, in a range of settings that was not shared by their able-bodied peers.

Despite growing legislative measures to prevent child labour, children with mental illnesses and disabilities clearly fulfilled economic roles throughout the period.[12] The value of their contribution is only just being revealed. It is difficult to offer firm explanations for why their economic role persisted, but it may have been that the mentally inferior child was simply not considered an innocent being in the same way as the mentally able. Furthermore, the labour of children in asylums was seen as therapeutic and a form of education, it was not an evil but a way of 'improving' and giving them some social value.[13] Such an approach subsequently made 'useless' children into productive beings, whether it was in the pauper lunatic asylum or on a Canadian farm.

In a social setting, the nature of the children and their behaviours have also been challenged. Cunningham argued that mischievousness was accepted as childhood exuberance by the end of the century, but in the case of children with mental health problems it was considered both a symptom and symbol of their mental inferiority.[14] The management of the mentally ill or disabled child in asylums, workhouses, schools, and their homes runs against the idea of childhood as a time of sheltered innocence for these individuals. The children were confined, labelled, and in extreme instances emigrated because of their failure to function normally or adhere to agreed social norms. Hardly the nostalgic childhood that our modern mentalities have come to conceptualise.

Looking more widely, the impact of social movements such as evangelicalism effected campaigns for the rights of the child, both in the home and workplace. Legislative changes such as the Factory Acts (1833–1878) and Education Acts (1870–1902) were considered successes for the reform movement and thought to crystallise the romantic idea of childhood. The evidence of child emigration fundamentally challenges the assumption of middle-class philanthropy working for the improvement of the child. The removal of insane children to far-away dominions of the empire forces us to reassess the impact that philanthropy had on conceptualising childhood. Clearly, very few children were subjected to a period of childhood innocence; they were thought a burden and removed to work on farms in Canada because of their impairment.

The narratives of emigrants, their settlement and embeddedness in new communities have all been topics of discussion in historical literature.[15] The experience of children and of settlement in Canada is largely overlooked. In the historiography of child emigration it appears that a re-evaluation of the types of children selected and the medical procedures they were subjected to is needed. The children that were part of this process were not the generic paupers that historians have assumed.[16] The consequences of such actions were wide-reaching and require a new approach to medical, social, and economic themes linked to the history of migration. Reconstructing the lives of these children, their experiences of working on farms, development into adulthood, and economic successes or failures as adults will enhance the histories of child insanity, migration, and settlement. It is clear that to understand the insanity of children in the era of asylums we have to look further than the walls of the institution and to the myriad of spaces that they occupied.

The experience of segregation provided specific issues for the Poor Law system. It has been argued that welfare provision was administered unevenly in nineteenth-century England and Wales with the north-west proving more parsimonious than the south-east.[17] A similar picture is true of the five asylums. The Prestwich Asylum was overcrowded and unwilling to accept children that could be managed in workhouses. Poor Law Guardians, however, were also reluctant to maintain children in the union. Such an aversion towards the care of these children meant that they were circulated through a network of welfare and medical provisions in the north-west. Up until now the experience of circulation through such a system has not been examined. At the heart of the problem was the question of who should pay for the care of insane children? Poor Law Guardians in the north-west argued that they should not be a burden to ratepayers and that central government should provide funds to pay for their care. Such attitudes go some way to explaining the involvement of mentally unsuitable children in the emigration programmes from this region during the late-nineteenth century. Conversely, the asylum in Northamptonshire benefited from the presence of child patients that had come from other county asylums. The development of a specialised children's block was intended to house children from outside the county at a higher rate than local patients. Through such an entrepreneurial approach the asylum in Northampton was able to become self-sufficient and not reliant on funds from the county. The welfare regimes of the north-west had very different experience of dealing with insane children than the authorities in Northamptonshire. Thus, there was a wider impact of insane children on the medical provisions of the Poor Law at local, regional, and national levels.

The treatment of pauper children also needs to be related to developments that affected Poor Law policy, independent of the asylum. The crusade against outdoor-relief during the late nineteenth century was particularly poignant. Elizabeth Hurren has shown that crusading policies reduced medical out-relief payments to families of the poor and in turn led to increased institutionalisation.[18] How children were affected by the crusade has not been explicitly examined. In 1869, at the outset of the crusade admissions of insane children peaked to voluntary hospitals, and then when at its peak in the mid-1880s the admission of children to asylums spiked. The reluctance of Guardians to pay out-relief to families led to the institutionalisation of more children who were likely to be a nuisance in the workhouse. Thus the removal of poor relief to help maintain the insane child in the domestic sphere placed additional strain on medical institutions of the time.

This book has exposed the complex nature of dealing with the mentally ill or disabled child. The implications affected not just the children themselves but also their families, communities, and authorities. Previously the insane child had not been located or placed in the historiography adequately and consequently the broader implications for their care and treatment had not been considered. The literature of asylums overlooks them, while the broader historical approaches of childhood, philanthropy, education, and emigration have not yet located their experiences or treatment. It is now clear that the insane child occupied a particular space in nineteenth-century England and their experiences to some extent have been identified.

Notes

1. NRO, St Crispin Collection, Female Casebook 8, NCLA6/2/1/8, Mabel Adkins, Admission no. 4003, p. 91.
2. BCA, All Saints Asylum, Male Casebook 14, MS344/12/14, Arthur Morecock, pp. 479–480.

3. A. Tanner, 'Choice and the Children's Hospital: Great Ormond Street Hospital and their Families 1855–1900,' in Borsay and Shapely (eds.), *Medicine, Charity and Mutual Aid: The Consumption of Health in Britain, c.1550–1950* (Ashgate: Oxon, 2007), pp. 135–162, p. 137.
4. A. Rebok Rosenthal, 'Insanity, Family and Community in Late-Victorian Britain,' in A. Borsay and P. Dale (eds.), *Disabled Children: Contested Caring, 1850–1979* (London: Pickering & Chatto, 2012), pp. 29–42; Melling et al., '"Proper Lunatic for Two Years": Pauper Lunatic Children in Victorian and Edwardian England. Child Admissions to the Devon County Lunatic Asylum, 1845–1914,' *Journal of Social History*, 31/2 (1997), pp. 371–405.
5. A. Scull, *Museums of Madness: The Social Organization of Insanity in Nineteenth-Century England* (London: Allen Lane, 1979); Scull, *The Most Solitary of Afflictions: Madness and Society in Britain 1700–1900* (London: Yale University Press, 1993).
6. Scull, *Museums of Madness*, pp. 240–248.
7. For a similar approach in the North Riding Asylum, Yorkshire, see R. Ellis, 'The Asylum, The Poor Law and the Growth of County Asylums in Nineteenth Century Yorkshire,' *Northern History*, 45/2 (2008), pp. 279–293.
8. S. Taylor, 'Insanity, Philanthropy and Emigration: Dealing with Insane Children in Late-Nineteenth-Century North-West England,' *History of Psychiatry*, 25/2 (2014), pp. 224–236.
9. LRO, Prestiwch Asylum, Female Casebook 3, GMCRO CHFC2/3, Ellen Ridings, Admission no. 6502, p. 425.
10. H. Cunningham, *Children and Childhood in Western Society since 1500* (London: Longman, 1995), p. 188.
11. J. Parr, *Labouring Children: British Immigrant Apprentices to Canada, 1869–1924* (London: Croom Helm, 1980).
12. J. Humphries, *Childhood and Child Labour in the British Industrial Revolution* (Cambridge, 2010); J. Humphries, 'Childhood and Child Labour in the British Industrial Revolution,' *The Economic History Review*, 66/2 (2013), pp. 395–418; P. Kirby, *Child Labour in Britain, 1750–1870* (London: Palgave, 2003), p. 131.
13. D. Wright, *Mental Disability in Victorian England: The Earlswood Asylum, 1847–1901* (Oxford: Clarendon, 2001).
14. Cunningham, *The Children of the Poor: Representations of Childhood since the Seventeenth Century* (Oxford: Blackwell, 1991), pp. 154–155.
15. D. Gerber, *Authors of their Own Lives: Personal Correspondence in the Lives of Nineteenth Century British Immigrants to the United States* (New York: New York University Press, 2006); D. Fitzpatrick, *Oceans of Consolation: Personal Accounts of Irish Migration to Australia* (Cork: Cork University

Press, 1995); M. Kleinig and E. Richards (eds.), *On the Wing: Mobility Before and After Emigration to Australia* (New South Wales: Anchor Books, 2013); E. Richards, *Destination Australia: Migration to Australia since 1901* (NSW: University of New South Wales Press, 2008); S. Sinke, *Dutch Immigrant Women in the United States, 1880–1920* (Champaign: University of Illinois Press, 2002); B. Elliot, D. Gerber, and S. Sinke (eds.), *Letters Across Borders: The Epistolary Practices of International Migrants* (Basingstoke: Palgrave Macmillan, 2006); T. Dublin (ed.), *Immigrant Voices: New Lives in America, 1773–1986* (Champaign: University of Illinois Press, 1993).

16. R. Parker, *Uprooted: The Shipment of Poor Children to Canada, 1867–1917* (Bristol: The Policy Press, 2008); L. Peters, *Orphan Texts: Victorian Orphans, Culture and Empire* (Manchester: Manchester University Press, 2000); J. Parr, *Labouring Children*; G. Wagner, *Children of the Empire* (London: Weidenfeld and Nicolson, 1982); P. Rooke and R. Schnell, 'Imperial Philanthropy and Colonial Response: British Juvenile Emigration to Canada, 1896–1930,' *The Historian*, 46/1 (1983), pp. 56–78; P. Bean and J. Melville, *Lost Children of the Empire* (London: Unwin Hyman, 1989); K. Bagnall, *The Little Immigrants: The Orphans who Came to Canada* (Toronto: Macmillan, 1989); M. Kohli, *The Golden Bridge: Young Immigrants to Canada, 1833–1939* (Toronto: National Heritage, 2003).
17. S. King, *Poverty and Welfare in England 1700–1850* (Manchester: Manchester University Press, 2000).
18. E. Hurren, *Protesting about Pauperism: Poverty, Politics and Poor Relief in Late-Victorian England, 1870–1900* (Woodbridge: Boydell & Brewer, 2008); Hurren, *Dying for Victorian Medicine: English Anatomy and its Trade in the Dead Poor* (Basingstoke: Palgrave Macmillan, 2011).

Index[1]

[1] Note: Page numbers followed by n denote footnotes

S.J. Taylor, *Child Insanity in England, 1845-1907*, Palgrave Studies in the History of Childhood, DOI 10.1007/978-1-137-60027-1

Printed in the United States
By Bookmasters